P160
1845
HJV DX ✓
(Hun)

Parasitic diseases in water resources development

The need for intersectoral negotiation

Books are to be returned on or before
the last date below.

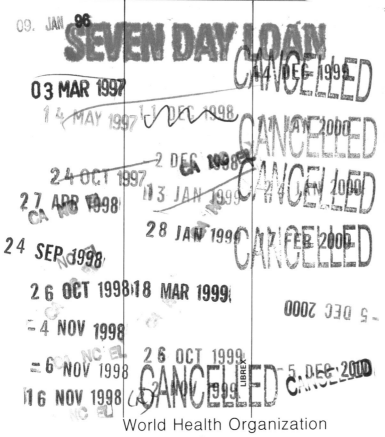

World Health Organization
Geneva
1993

9241561556

WHO Library Cataloguing in Publication Data

Parasitic diseases in water resources development : the
    need for intersectoral negotiation / J. M. Hunter. . .
    [et al.]

1.Disease vectors   2.Health policy   3.Parasitic diseases –
prevention & control   4.Water resources development
I. Hunter, J. M.

ISBN 92 4 156155 6   (NLM Classification: WC 695)

Typeset in India
Printed in England

91/9105 – Macmillans/Clays/Mosaic – 8000

Contents

Preface

One of the cornerstones of WHO's Global Strategy for Health for All by the Year 2000 is intersectoral collaboration, and various resolutions of the World Health Assembly have encouraged WHO and its Member States to promote such collaboration in order to address the health aspects of development policies.

The increased awareness of the environment, together with the feasibility of controlling parasitic diseases, provides a good opportunity to focus attention on the health impact of development. Several such diseases can be exacerbated by water development projects unless appropriate measures for prevention and control are incorporated from the beginning. The health sector therefore needs to be involved at every stage of such projects in order to ensure that socioeconomic development does not bring about a deterioration in health status.

This book reviews the documented health impact of various water resources development projects and discusses the actions that could have mitigated the adverse effects. The message derived from the analysis is that sound proposals to control parasitic diseases could and should have been included in the development dialogue. For this to occur, the health sector needs to take a much more active role in ensuring that other sectors are aware of the potential health impact of development projects.

The analysis given here is of necessity incomplete and with a bias related to the ease of availability of data. The documentation of negative effects is not intended to be a deterrent to development. Rather it is hoped that it will encourage more complete and systematic monitoring of the health effects of water resources development, and provide a guide to the risks to be considered and the input needed from the health sector.

Readers are invited to send any information, comments or suggestions related to this publication to Chief, Schistosomiasis and other Trematode Infections, Division of Control of Tropical Diseases, World Health Organization, 1211 Geneva 27, Switzerland.

Acknowledgements

Our appreciation and sincere thanks go to Mr R. Bos, Secretary of the FAO/UNEP/WHO Panel of Experts on Environmental Management; Dr R. Goodland, Chief, Department of Environment, World Bank, Washington, DC, USA; Ms Catherine Mulholland, Assistant to the Adviser on Health and Development Policies, Office of the Director-General, WHO; and Dr S. Litsios, Operational Research, Division of Control of Tropical Diseases, WHO, who provided detailed written critiques of the draft document and additional materials without which it would not have been possible to clarify the most difficult issues on contemporary development policy.

We are also grateful for the documentation and expert opinion freely given by the following WHO staff members: Dr P. F. Beales, Chief, Training, Division of Control of Tropical Diseases; Dr A. El Bindari Hammad, Adviser on Health and Development Policies; Dr P. Herath, Scientist, Operational Research, Division of Control of Tropical Diseases; Dr R. Leberre, Chief, Filariasis Control, Division of Control of Tropical Diseases; and Mr H. Dixon, Chief, Epidemiology and Statistical Methodology, Division of Epidemiological Surveillance and Health Situation and Trend Assessment.

Many of the documents prepared for the WHO Informal Meeting on the Global Strategy for the Control of Morbidity due to Schistosomiasis, held in October 1989 and supported by the Edna McConnell Clark Foundation, were useful in the preparation of this document. All the WHO Regional Advisers on Parasitic Diseases commented on and contributed to the draft manuscript.

The following people kindly supplied valuable information, mostly based on field observations:

Dr M. A. Amin, Ministry of Health, Gizan, Saudi Arabia; Professor F. Arfaa, Concord, California, USA; Dr F. S. Barbosa, Dean, National School of Public Health, Rio de Janeiro, Brazil; Dr D. J. Bradley, London School of Hygiene and Tropical Medicine, London, England; Dr C. A. Brown, Bureau of Hygiene and Tropical Disease, London, England;

Dr J. Cook, Edna McConnell Clark Foundation, New York, USA; Dr M. Delabaere, "Prince Léopold" Institute, Antwerp, Belgium; Dr A. Gani, Ministry of Health, Depok, Indonesia; Professor E. G. Garcia, School of Public Health, University of the Philippines, Manila, Philippines; Dr P. L. Gigase, Laboratory of Histopathology and Schistosomiasis, "Prince Léopold" Institute, Antwerp, Belgium; Dr S. M. El Hak, Ministry of Health, Cairo, Egypt; Dr L. Iarotski, Martsinovsky Institute of Medical Parasitology, Moscow, Russian Federation; Dr W. R. Jobin, Blue Nile Associates, Foxboro, Massachusetts, USA; Dr P. Jordan, Ware, England; Professor M. Le Bras, Department of Health and Development, University of Bordeaux II, Bordeaux, France; Professor Madya Pheng Kan Chua, Department of Parasitology, Faculty of Medicine, Kuala Lumpur, Malaysia; Dr E. A. Malek, Director, Laboratory of Schistosomiasis, Medical Center, New Orleans, USA; Professor S. P. Mao, Director, Institute of Parasitic Diseases, Chinese Academy of Preventive Medicine, Shanghai, China; Dr D. A. Muir, Geneva, Switzerland; Dr A. S. Muller, Director, Department of Tropical Hygiene, Royal Tropical Institute, Amsterdam, Netherlands; Dr M. Odei, Institute of Aquatic Biology, Achimota, Ghana; Dr J. L. Rey, Department of Epidemiology, French Institute for Cooperative Scientific Research for Development (ORSTOM), Abidjan, Côte d'Ivoire; Dr H. P. Striebel, Ciba-Geigy, Basel, Switzerland; Dr T. I. Soewarso, Ministry of Health, Jakarta, Indonesia; Dr V. R. Southgate, Experimental Taxonomy Unit, Department of Zoology, British Museum, London, England; Dr R. F. Sturrock, Department of Medical Helminthology, London School of Hygiene and Tropical Medicine, St Albans, England; Professor H. Tanaka, Public Health Laboratory of Chiba Prefecture, Chiba, Japan; Dr P. G. Waiyaki, Kenya Medical Research Institute, Nairobi, Kenya: Dr K. S. Warren, Maxwell Communications, New York, USA; Professor G. Webbe, Winches Farm, London School of Hygiene and Tropical Medicine, St Albans, England; and Dr F. Wurapa, WHO Regional Office for Africa, Brazzaville, Congo.

We are grateful to Miss J. Salm and Miss J. Mercado for typing the manuscript under pressure of tight deadlines.

1.
Introduction

The development of water resources is essential for a wide range of human activities. In particular it is needed so that demands for energy and food can be met. However, during the past ten years, certain adverse effects of water resources development have received considerable attention. The rate of population growth in developing countries continues to outstrip their capacity to meet the demands for food and basic services amid increasing poverty. The prospect of environmental degradation in the face of development was examined by the World Commission on Environment and Development (1987). The health impact of this degradation was emphasized in the report of the WHO Commission on Health and Environment, *Our planet, our health* (WHO, 1992a). This report contributed significantly to the debate on the impact of development on the environment and health at the Earth Summit, the United Nations Conference on Environment and Development, held in Rio de Janeiro in June 1992.

Development policies designed to improve the economic conditions and living standards of communities often have unintended effects on health (Cooper Weil et al., 1990). Thus, health policy is not a matter solely for the health sector, and it is now accepted that there should be health objectives in water resources development. Furthermore, the identification of vulnerable groups and their health risks is necessary so that adverse socioeconomic factors can be combated.

Awareness of the negative health effects of development, particularly in respect of parasitic diseases, has not led to consistent action either in the planning stages of projects or at the first signs of unfavourable consequences. During the 1970s, the public began to appreciate that economic development could produce adverse effects on human health, as pointed out by Hughes & Hunter (1970). Since then the epidemiological factors contributing to the introduction, spread or aggravation of parasitic diseases have become more fully understood. There have been advances in diagnosis and treatment, and options for community-based health care delivery have become available. Moreover, the connections between health, environment and development have become clearer. The inadequacy of data on the link between economic

1

considerations and environmental events cannot excuse a failure to reckon with the available health data. The underlying causes of poor health may be activities that seem remote from the observed effects. The focus of this book is justified by the significant amount of data available, the impact of parasitic diseases on people involved in or living near water resources projects, and the feasibility of mitigating, preventing and controlling these diseases.

It is now recognized that measures of mitigation and prevention should be a shared responsibility in the development process. Donors and entrepreneurs in developed countries can no longer claim ignorance of the potential negative health outcomes, nor can governments of developing countries justify the ecological changes inherent in water resources development on purely economic grounds. More importantly, the political will of developing countries to address these problems is now a matter of public record. The incidence and prevalence of parasitic diseases and certain other communicable diseases remain the most dramatic and reliable indicators of the negative health impacts of development in Africa, Asia and the Americas.

In earlier reviews, evidence was assembled to show the adverse disease impact caused by water resources development (Ackermann et al., 1973; Stanley & Alpers, 1975; Hunter et al., 1980, 1982). Action without consultation by different sectors was identified as the main factor engendering disregard and neglect of human health. A policy of integrated project development was offered, with carefully planned support for health maintenance in and around large reservoirs and irrigation systems.

Today, with a population doubling time of 34 years in the developing world, the need for dams and irrigation schemes is greater than ever before. In the 1970s the economic justification for constructing reservoirs began to be questioned (UNEP, 1982). The economic and nutritional justifications for expanding agriculture and irrigation remain paramount (Lipton & de Kadt, 1988), while there has been a public and political awakening to environmental problems (UNEP, 1987a, 1988, 1989, 1990). Aside from visible degradation, disease in exposed populations may be the first consequence that provokes public reaction. Despite this, adverse health effects of water resources development continue unabated (Service, 1989a,b).

Health officials in developing countries need to enter the development dialogue to place health on the national development agenda. The obvious arguments for entering the dialogue may be the impetus required to induce action at the higher levels of government. While it may appear that intersectoral dialogue in the international or multilateral arenas can be achieved, its success in practice and the impact on health are questioned by the studies documented in this book. The lack of dialogue and its inevitable outcome—lack of action—are predictable.

Those who understand health problems and, as the case in point, parasitic diseases, those who assess the results of intervention, and those who propose solutions move independently of those who decide and implement water resources development projects. Lack of foresight, the adverse consequences, and their late recognition are the fruit of this continuing lack of communication.

The global agenda on environmental issues now includes health (UNEP, 1986, 1990; WHO, 1992a; World Bank/International Monetary Fund, 1989). The international development finance community endorses environmental impact assessment through more integrated and health-conscious planning. Speedier change and more resolute commitment to health protection are needed. The present analysis is intended to promote the movement towards more integrated development activities, incorporating health protection and promotion measures along with economic advancement. Evidence concerning water-related parasitic diseases is reviewed in a broad policy context. Detailed information on other communicable diseases or health problems that may affect specific regions, such as dengue and Japanese encephalitis, may be found elsewhere. An exposition of associations between disease and environment is followed by an outline of the adverse health effects of dams and irrigation systems. The need is emphasized for continuing vigilance as water-related development proceeds on a massive scale. Small dams are presented as a special case in Chapter 4. The current status of technical measures for disease control is summarized in Chapter 5.

A policy critique (Chapter 6) is followed by proposed practical steps towards solutions. If the tools described are used, the best possible terms for health should be obtainable. Intersectoral negotiating strategies for health officials are considered in Chapter 8, and finally, the preparation of a health plan for a water resources project is outlined.

2.

Parasitic diseases and water resources development

Exacerbation of parasitic diseases

Outstanding among the parasitic diseases exacerbated by water resources development projects are lymphatic filariasis, malaria and schistosomiasis. Although the importance of lymphatic filariasis is widely recognized among health workers, the onset and increase of the disease in these situations are poorly documented. This presents a major challenge for the future monitoring of parasitic diseases in water resources development.

The present book concentrates on four parasitic diseases—malaria, schistosomiasis, lymphatic filariasis and onchocerciasis—but this should not be interpreted as indicating that they are the only ones of concern in water resources projects. There is a plethora of guidelines on potential health risks, with no analysis of cause-and-effect relationships or documentation of effective mitigation or intervention, which is of little use to planners or actors on the health scene. Water resources projects lead to the aggregation of people; the ensuing health consequences include sexually transmitted diseases, accidental injuries, acute respiratory infections, diarrhoea and tuberculosis. In the earliest phases of water resources planning, it is imperative to undertake a systematic review and to establish a priority ranking for the prevention and control of all health risks.

Parasitic infections caused by protozoa, such as African trypanosomiasis, Chagas disease, and cutaneous and visceral leishmaniasis, have geographical specificity. The effects on nutritional status and health of the ubiquitous intestinal helminths (*Ascaris,* hookworm and *Trichuris*) and protozoa (*Amoeba, Giardia* and *Cryptosporidia*) should not be ignored, since there are effective strategies of prevention and control (WHO, 1987c; Pawlowski et al., 1991).

The omission of reference to viral infections, which apart from hepatitis B are focal or geographically specific, is intentional. The occurrence of Japanese encephalitis has been closely associated with rice fields. This disease has created serious public health problems in India, Indonesia, the Republic of Korea, Sri Lanka, and some states of the former USSR. It appears to be

4

subsiding in China, Japan, and the Republic of Korea but is spreading in Bangladesh, India, Myanmar, Nepal, Thailand and Viet Nam (Umenai et al., 1985). Increases in incidence and distribution have been attributed to the switch from dry-land to irrigated rice cultivation and to the establishment of large modern pig farms. This disease is being reduced in several countries through immunization programmes and the control of the mosquito vector.

Sylvatic yellow fever in Brazil and West Africa is not a serious health problem, thanks to efficient vaccination coverage of the people at risk in water resources projects. The known distribution of the mosquito vectors of dengue, o'nyong nyong (in Kenya), and other arboviral diseases permits the prediction of risk in water development projects (Adekolu-John & Fagbami, 1980).

Ecological disruption at project sites

The construction of dams and formation of reservoirs and irrigation systems in tropical areas can cause rapid environmental degradation, and health risks may arise even before there is any awareness of the danger and before preparations have been made to overcome it (Burgis & Morris, 1987; Carpenter, 1987; Payne, 1986).

Every lake undergoes an evolution that gradually leads to its basin being filled up. Impounded lakes are subject to this process and their useful life can be predicted. It could be 500 years as in Lake Nasser, or less than 100 years as for many small dams. Watershed abuse leading to silting can reduce the life of a dam by more than half. Changes in the characteristics of the ecosystem represented by an artificial lake and the territory exposed to its influence occur more rapidly. In the first instance there are changes due to water retention: the flooding of territory, the rise in the groundwater level, the submersion of the terrestrial flora and fauna, and the forced departure of people and animals.

There are also gradual changes due to the accumulation of chemical products derived from the carbon, calcium, magnesium, nitrogen and phosphorus cycles that convert the ecosystem from an oligotrophic status with low nutrient concentrations to a eutrophic status, characterized by a richness of nutrients, a high density of certain populations, a very high biological oxygen demand, and a reduced number of species able to survive under these conditions. The surface of the water may acquire so much floating vegetation that fishing, navigation and even the passage of small boats become impossible. The accumulation of organic matter at the bottom and the consumption of oxygen for its oxidation eventually produce a zone where aerobic flora and fauna cannot exist. The fermentation of masses of dead algae and other

5

organisms sometimes causes such pronounced changes in the quality of the water that it becomes unsuitable for human purposes.

Efforts should be made to conserve the good qualities of water, not only for domestic use but also for the maintenance of a biological equilibrium compatible with fish farming, the control of floating and riverside vegetation, and other requirements. If an undertaking is to function as planned with turbines, irrigation, navigation, fishing and recreation, thorough knowledge and continuing surveillance of environmental conditions are required.

Changes in surrounding areas

Water resources development does not occur in isolation. The construction of a dam creates changes in both the upstream and downstream areas.

The initial concern is for the sources of the rivers feeding the lake, because it is often there that environmental degradation commences as a result of forest clearance, which is likely to be followed by a reduction or drying up of watercourses.

In forests, part of the rainwater returns to the atmosphere by evaporation, some is retained by the vegetation, and part is absorbed by the ground. Forest clearance upsets this balance, especially in humid tropical climates where the removal of plant cover leads to intense erosion and loss of soil fertility. The flow of rivers becomes irregular; rapid rainwater run-off causes floods and, during low-rainfall periods, streams may dry up or become blocked by sand deposits. This has both direct and indirect repercussions on the health of riverside populations, especially in poor countries. Swamps and pools, even if they exist for only a short time after flooding, become breeding places for blood-sucking insect vectors of disease and for snails that act as intermediate hosts.

Deforestation and erosion favour the rapid deposition of sediments and dissolved substances, especially if fertilizers and other chemical products are used in cultivated fields. The eutrophication of lakes is accelerated and species diversity is reduced.

In a few impounded lakes, forest flooding has, in the short term, resulted in enriched fish production. This is attributed to the response of plankton to the abundance of organic matter. In Africa, similar situations have encouraged fishing and populations have moved towards lakes where, because of more frequent contact with water containing *Biomphalaria* or *Bulinus* snails, the transmission of schistosomiasis has become more intense. Since the very favourable conditions of fish harvesting are short-lived, the economic status of these communities gradually deteriorates, and health conditions worsen if special measures are not taken.

In the downstream area, irrigated agriculture greatly simplifies the landscape and reduces the diversity of the fauna and flora.

Other changes accompanying this type of agricultural exploitation are: an increase in the area covered by water; the development of swampy regions and lagoons on surrounding terrain lower than the lake or on the fringes of cultivated land, as a result of the rise in the groundwater level; and some modification of the microclimate, with generally more constant humidity throughout the year and increased insolation.

Depending on their ecology, certain mosquito species may disappear or remain confined to small territories untouched by development. Other species may find more favourable conditions: increased water surface; favourable physical, chemical or nutritional factors in lakes, irrigation canals, excavations, marshes and seepage zones; and reduced numbers of predators, allowing the vectors' abundance to increase and enhancing their ability to transmit diseases. Both the extension of the aquatic habitat and the state of the ecosystem at a certain stage of eutrophication may favour the establishment or multiplication of snail species acting as intermediate hosts for schistosomes or other trematodes.

In tropical lakes the extraordinary growth of certain species of floating plants, particularly *Eichhornia crassipes* (water hyacinth), *Salvinia auriculata* (water fern) and *Pistia stratiotes* (water lettuce), provides rich support for the multiplication of important vector snails, especially *Bulinus* and *Biomphalaria* species, and of insects. Moreover, snail dispersal along watercourses is assisted by floating islets of vegetation. The spread of water hyacinth is having a severe economic impact on Lake Victoria, Lake Kyoga, and the Nile river source in Uganda. Submerged vegetation, of which *Ceratophyllum demersum*, *Polygonum senegalense* and *Utricularia inflexa* are examples, may support large snail colonies, especially when the aquatic plants are growing vigorously. Sometimes, as occurred in Lake Nasser, bottom algae can support a snail population that ensures the transmission of schistosomiasis.

Population movement and socioeconomic and demographic change

From the public health viewpoint, the new ecological conditions and their repercussions on the vectors and mechanisms of disease transmission take on their full significance in relation to socioeconomic and demographic changes occurring simultaneously (Goldsmith & Hildyard, 1985, 1986).

The original occupants of a flooded region have to bear the consequences of the abandonment of crops, field sites, and homes, and the reorganization of their lives. This is stressful even if new properties, dwellings and economic resources are offered to them (Roundy, 1989). Almost 100 000 people were displaced from the Bandama valley in Côte d'Ivoire when Lake Kossou was created, and the same fate befell about 65 000 in the Itaipu basin of Brazil and Uruguay. Estimates of the number of people likely to be displaced by the Narmada Valley Project in India vary from 300 000 to a million. Such upheavals risk exposing people, especially children and the aged, to exceptional adversities in the areas of nutrition, housing and hygiene, at a time when health risks are elevated, possibly as a consequence of rehousing on the shores of a lake or in an irrigation zone where there is increased vector density and contact with new immigrants.

Furthermore, workers involved in the construction of dams and irrigation networks, and their families, sometimes come from distant regions and may affect the epidemiological situation as follows:

— by introducing diseases;
— by introducing new strains of a parasite or new vectors, possibly better adapted than the original ones to the ecological conditions that have been created;
— by lacking immunity to local pathogens;
— by increasing the population density in the foci of transmission.

Reservoirs and irrigation systems are often sited in regions where only animal production or subsistence farming existed previously. New types of activity become available to the population: construction, fishing or agricultural work involving new techniques and, often, more contact with water, pesticides and chemical fertilizers.

Conversely, immigrant workers and technicians from urban centres are brought into direct contact with ecological niches where there are sylvatic or rural diseases of which they have no experience, such as yellow fever, leishmaniasis, trypanosomiasis, malaria and filariasis.

Nosological and epidemiological changes

Diseases already present

Ecological changes can modify the incidence and prevalence of diseases already present in a region. These will tend to decrease if, for example, specific vectors or those playing the most effective role in transmission are reduced. The destruction of primeval forests in Brazil reduces the population of the sandfly species that is mainly responsible for the propagation of cutaneous leishmaniasis. After an increase in the incidence of leishmaniasis following first contact with the forest, a change is observed as the trees are destroyed or submerged, new cases become rarer and the disease finally disappears.

It is generally accepted that the risk of African trypanosomiasis or sleeping sickness in water resources developments in areas of known endemicity decreases rather than increases (Finelle, 1980), since the vector, *Glossina*, breeds only on seasonally or permanently dry soil. It has been suggested, but never confirmed, that some sites of taro cultivation with swamp irrigation in Nigeria and of rice irrigation in Gambia were associated with increased *Glossina* populations. The observation by Finelle (1980) that sugar cane irrigation in Côte d'Ivoire was associated with increased numbers of cases of sleeping sickness can possibly be explained by the proximity of the irrigation system to the forest breeding sites of *Glossina* rather than by breeding sites within the scheme itself or the presence of infected migrant workers, as occurred in a sugar plantation at Mbandjock, Cameroon (Eouzan, 1980). This illustrates the importance of the siting of water resources projects and of the surrounding environment (Mbulamberi, 1989).

Similarly, the inundation of breeding sites of *Simulium* effectively eliminates transmission of onchocerciasis. On the other hand, if inundation is caused by a dam, both the spillways and the downstream rapids may become ideal breeding sites for the insects.

Usually, however, there is a tendency towards increased incidence or prevalence of malaria and schistosomiasis. In South America the multiplication of malaria mosquitos *(Anopheles darlingi, A. pseudopunctipennis* and *A. albimanus)* is favoured by the construction of dams and irrigation networks. *A. albimanus* also transmits arboviruses. In different phases of rice cultivation a succession of mosquito species may appear throughout the year.

Culex tarsalis, very characteristic of irrigated regions, is an important vector of St Louis encephalitis. In California more than 80% of the breeding places of mosquitos responsible for annual outbreaks of encephalitis are man-made.

Impounded lakes, and irrigation canals to an even greater extent, generally provide highly favourable habitats for aquatic snails. Densities of *Biomphalaria* and *Bulinus* become much greater in these man-made environments than in the original breeding places (Andrade, 1969; Coumbaras & Picot, 1979). At the same time, human contacts with the water increase through activities such as fishing, irrigation and canal maintenance, or because of people's domestic needs where housing and environmental sanitation are unsatisfactory.

In water development projects generally there is a great variety of environmental and settlement conditions and consequently of disease risks (Roundy, 1989).

Disease occurring during the construction phase

A wide range of health problems may arise during construction especially diseases that are directly related to man-made lakes but not waterborne.

Predisposing conditions are created by the arrival of large numbers of workers to engage in temporary activities. In Itaipu, Brazil, where up to 38 000 people were employed on dam construction, the turnover at the end of 1978 was around 2000 departures or arrivals a day. The incoming workers and their families increased the population of nearby villages 3–7-fold. Living mostly in overcrowded slums with neither sanitation nor adequate health care, they were exposed to the common infectious diseases, particularly respiratory and diarrhoeal infections, malnutrition and polyparasitism, leading to impaired development of children. The living conditions were also conducive to prostitution and promiscuity, with a high frequency of sexually transmitted diseases (SUCAM, 1976).

At construction sites, occupational diseases and accidents at work are to be expected. In Itaipu there were 8.4 accidents per 100 000 work-hours, and 10% of the workers each year required sick leave (Brasil-Paraguay Itaipu Binacional, 1978; Rey, 1978). In Salto Grande, on the Argentina-Uruguay border, between June 1974 and March 1980, there were 17 construction deaths and an accident rate of 0.91 per employee per year.

Diseases appearing after project completion

Ecosystem changes around large water projects may favour the introduction of parasitic diseases not previously reported and their recognition may be delayed for years after schemes have been completed. Intermediate snail hosts may be introduced by fishermen, farm workers, or domestic animals, and even by birds. The primary introduction of mosquito vectors of malaria and filariasis and the initiation of transmission by them remains to be documented.

In some cases what seems to be a recrudescence of a local disease may be a new problem transplanted from elsewhere. The outbreak of schistosomiasis at Lake Volta is a good example. In the rivers of the region where the lake was formed there was a strain of *Schistosoma haematobium* transmitted by *Bulinus globosus* and responsible for a low endemicity among the local Krobo people. *Bu. globosus* never succeeded in establishing itself in the new lake but Ewe fishermen, coming from coastal lagoons, introduced *Bulinus truncatus rohlfsi* into the new habitat. The Ewe also brought a new strain of *S. haematobium* to the shores of the lake; the larval part of its cycle takes place in *Bu. truncatus rohlfsi* but is unable to infect *Bu. globosus*. Studies by Chu et al. (1981) have shown that the *Schistosoma* strain transmitted by *Bu. globosus* does not develop in *Bu. truncatus*, and thus we are confronted by two forms of schistosomiasis, linked to two different ecosystems, the first autochthonous and the second arriving after the creation of Lake Volta and being responsible for high endemic prevalence along its shores.

Need for water resources development

World population increase

World population expansion can be considered as having two separate stages. The first, from 1750 to 1950, was triggered by the Industrial Revolution, when rapid growth rates occurred in Europe, the Americas and Oceania where Europeans settled. The second began about 1950 with growth occurring mainly in developing countries, as a result of reduced death rates, improved standards of living, better public health, and the continuation of high birth rates.

The highest growth rates are currently in Africa and Latin America, which are expected to increase their share of world population from 15.5% in 1950 to 23.1% in 2000 (Table 1). The population of developing countries increased 2.2 times from 1950 to 1985 and is expected to be 2.9 times greater than in 1950 by the year 2000. For Latin America and Africa the corresponding increases are expected to be 3.3 and 3.9 times.

Economic growth and food needs

To satisfy the needs of these fast-growing populations, food production will have to follow the same trend. According to the Food and Agriculture Organization of the United Nations, using an index of 100 for 1979–81,

Table 1. Estimated population growth until the year 2100 in developing countries and percentages of world population

Year	Latin America[a]		Africa		Developing regions[b]	
	Millions	**%**	**Millions**	**%**	**Millions**	**%**
1950	165	6.6	224	8.9	1681	66.8
1985	405	8.4	555	11.5	3657	75.6
2000	546	8.9	872	14.2	4837	79.0
2025	779	9.5	1617	19.7	6799	82.9
2100	1238	12.2	2591	25.4	8748	85.9

Source: World Resources Institute, 1987.
[a] Including Mexico and the Caribbean.
[b] Including Latin America, Africa and Asia, except Japan.

world food production increased from 70 in 1964–66 to 110 in 1983–85; but per capita production rose from 94 to only 102 during the same period.

In Africa, food production increased in this period from 71 to 109, but per capita production declined from 108 to 96. In South America it rose from 64 to 107 while the per capita value rose from 91 to 98. Some Central American countries had better per capita results, namely Costa Rica (77 to 90), Cuba (70 to 108), Dominican Republic (94 to 105), Jamaica (91 to 103), and Mexico (90 to 99).

In Africa and Asia almost all agricultural land is farmed in smallholdings of less than 5 ha (50 000 m^2) or medium-sized holdings ranging from 5 to 50 ha. Most holdings in Latin America are small, but the majority of the agricultural area is farmed in larger holdings exceeding 50 ha. Many small-holdings occupy marginal land and tend to shrink because of land scarcity and

Table 2. Irrigated areas in some countries of Africa and Latin America, 1988, and percentage change from 1973 to 1988

Country	Area irrigated in 1988 (1000s of ha)	Percentage change, 1973–88
Africa	11 146	17
Algeria	365	34
Egypt	2 580	− 11
Libyan Arab Jamahiriya	240	21
Madagascar	890	56
Mali	205	54
Morocco	1 260	20
Nigeria	860	6
Sudan	1 880	11
Tunisia	280	63
Latin America	15 642	27
Argentina	1 740	21
Brazil	2 600	58
Chile	1 260	2
Colombia	510	45
Cuba	870	39
Ecuador	547	12
Guyana	130	8
Mexico	5 100	19
Peru	1 240	10
Suriname	31	46
Venezuela	290	12

Source: FAO (1989b).

population pressure. In Brazil, however, the average size of smallholdings has increased because new agricultural land has been created by the clearance of forests.

When arable land becomes scarce, increases in agricultural production have to be obtained by gaining better yields. This is achieved through irrigation, improved seed varieties, mechanization, the use of fertilizers and pesticides, and other inputs (Table 2). Over 40% of the world's crops are produced on irrigated land, which represents 15% of the arable area.

Rate of construction of dams

Dams, irrigation systems and freshwater fisheries are indicators of the development process. The rate at which they are built in a country may outstrip the capacity of the health care system to monitor the introduction, spread or aggravation of parasitic diseases. Since most of these projects do not have an adequate health component, the magnitude of the problem can only be understood in terms of their rate of growth.

Global overview

According to the International Commission on Large Dams (ICOLD, 1989), there were 5270 dams in 1950; from 1951 to 1977, an average of 357 dams were constructed per year; for 1978 to 1982, the corresponding figure was 335 dams annually, and for 1983 to 1986, it was 209 dams per year. Approximately half the dams are in China, which has 18 800, the rest of the world having 17 400.

Three "megadams", with reservoir surfaces exceeding 1000 km^2, existed before 1950; eight were built between 1950 and 1959; 21 were constructed between 1960 and 1969 (Fels & Keller, 1973), and 15 from 1970 to 1986. Lake Volta, covering 8500 km^2, and with a 5000 km shore-line, is the world's largest man-made impoundment.

Small dams, below 15 metres in height, are far more numerous and are closely linked with agricultural activities. The construction of small dams, advocated by the international financing community as a manageable and practical solution to land and water conservation, has been facilitated by the easier access to and purchase of bulldozers – the so-called "bulldozer revolution".

At the last reckoning there were 423 dams in Africa (excluding South Africa) over 10 m high, 1487 in Latin America, and 3543 in Asia (excluding Japan) (Tables 3–6). The trend observed in almost all developing countries is to increase land productivity through water storage and irrigation projects.

The number of large dams constructed for irrigation and hydroelectric energy seems to be limited only by the availability of investment. Geographically, substantial potential exists for the conversion of moving water into electricity. In 1985, dams accounted for about 6.7% of the world's primary energy, and the World Energy Conference has projected that hydropower will supply six times the current output by 2020.

Two-thirds of the unexploited hydropower potential lies in developing countries. While Europe uses 59% of its exploitable potential, and North America 36%, developing countries utilize only 7%. Brazil, China, Colombia, India, Peru and Zaire have the largest untapped potential. The great river basins, such as those of the Amazon, Congo and Mekong, have yet to be developed.

Dams in Africa

Water impoundment schemes can be graded as large, medium or small, using either the classification of the Knoxville International Symposium on Man-Made Lakes (Ackermann, White & Worthington, 1973) or that of the International Commission on Large Dams (ICOLD, 1973, 1985, 1989).

Information on national construction programmes is easier to obtain for large and medium impoundments than for small dams; the large impoundments are fewer, they require central funds and other resources, and often have a national objective, while small dams generally derive from local needs, decisions and inputs.

During the 1960s and 1970s, 202 large dams were built in Africa; in the 1980s, 131 more were added (Table 3). New impoundments have been proposed in Algeria, Côte d'Ivoire, Ghana, Morocco and Nigeria, and many are already under construction. In 1977, Nigeria allocated 10 million naira (approximately US$ 17 500 000) for feasibility studies and engineering design for proposed dams and irrigation schemes in nine river basins. In the Sudan a large new irrigation system, the Rahad, has been developed and further extensions to the irrigation system of the Gezira are planned.

The major African dams are listed in Table 4, where it can be seen that many were built during the 1980s. Zimbabwe is a good example of a country with a solid infrastructure and the ability to expand even further. Its first dam was constructed in 1901, and before 1940 there were five; during the 1940s another five were added, and in the succeeding decades, 8, 21, 33 and 29 were constructed, giving a total of 101 dams (ICOLD, 1989).

In Kenya there has recently been highly intensive development of water resources in a single hydrological area, the Tana Basin. In 1968 the Kindruma Dam, 24 m high, was completed (Vogel et al., 1974). It was followed in rapid

14

Table 3. Number of dams over 10 m high built in Africa (excluding South Africa)

Country	Before 1961	1961–80	After 1980[a]
Algeria	15	6	22
Angola	3	7	5
Benin	–	1	1
Botswana	–	3	–
Burkina Faso	–	1	1
Cameroon	1	5	3
Congo	1	1	–
Côte d'Ivoire	1	18	3
Egypt	4	1	–
Ethiopia	3	5	–
Gabon	–	1	–
Ghana	–	4	1
Guinea	–	2	–
Kenya	2	5	7
Lesotho	–	2	1
Liberia	–	1	–
Libyan Arab Jamahiriya	–	8	4
Madagascar	8	2	–
Malawi	2	1	–
Mali	–	–	2
Mauritius	2	3	1
Morocco	13	14	35
Mozambique	1	4	3
Nigeria	2	34	9
Senegal	–	–	2
Sierra Leone	–	1	–
Sudan	2	2	–
Swaziland	–	5	1
Togo	–	1	1
Uganda	1	–	–
United Republic of Tanzania	–	2	–
Zaire	7	7	1
Zambia	2	2	–
Zimbabwe	20	53	28
Total	90	202	131

Source: ICOLD, 1989.
[a] Completed or under construction.

succession by the Kamburu (1974, 56 m), Gitaru (1978, 30 m), Masinga (1980, 70 m) and Kiambere (1988, 112 m) Dams, the last still being under construction. Such a staircase of five large dams brings fundamental ecological changes in addition to increased levels of schistosomiasis.

Table 4. Dates of construction of representative major dams in Africa

Dam (country and river)	Date of completion
Aswan Low Dam (Egypt, Nile)	1933
Owen Falls (Uganda, White Nile)	1954
Kariba (Zambia/Zimbabwe, Zambezi)	1959
Akosombo (Ghana, Volta)	1964
Kainji (Nigeria, Niger)	1968
Aswan High Dam (Egypt/Sudan, Nile)	1970
Kafue (Zambia, Kafue)	1971
Kossou (Côte d'Ivoire, Bandama)	1972
Cabora Bassa (Mozambique, Zambezi)	1974
Kamburu (Kenya, Tana)	1975
Legadadi (Ethiopia, Sendafa)	1979
Masinga (Kenya, Tana)	1980
Kpong (Ghana, Volta)	1981
Selingue (Mali, Sankaran)	1982
Shioro (Nigeria, Kaduna/Dinya)	1984
Diama (Senegal, Senegal/St Louis)	1986
Nangbeto (Benin, Mono)	1987[a]
Kompienga (Burkina Faso, Kompienga)	1988[a]
Manantali (Mali/Senegal, Senegal)	1988[a]
Capanda (Angola, Cuanza)	1992[a]

Source: ICOLD, 1989.
[a] Under construction or delayed.

Dams in the Americas

The number of artificial lakes in Latin America is continually increasing (Table 5). In Brazil an estimated hydroelectric potential of 80 000 MW is now tapped through the activity of more than 400 hydroelectric plants. Two new giant plants have been constructed: Itaipu (12 600 MW) on the Paraná River and Tucurui (8000 MW) on the Tocantins River. Some ten major lakes are being created annually. On the frontier between Argentina and Uruguay (Uruguay River) there is a big hydroelectric plant at Salto Grande; another is under construction between Argentina and Paraguay (Paraná River) at Yacyretá.

Numerous small and medium-sized impoundments, some 800 of them in north-east Brazil, have been built for irrigation or other purposes. The creation of new dams seems endless as the cultivated area expands and agricultural technology is improved.

In Venezuela in 1976 there were 54 artificial lakes, four were under construction and eight others were planned. Irrigated areas amounted to 64 914 ha in 1968 and 74 251 ha in 1972; during 1973, about 5000 ha of

Table 5. Number of dams over 10 m high built in Latin America

Country	Before 1950	1951–60	1961–70	1971–80	After 1980[a]	Total
Argentina	22	15	16	30	17	100
Bolivia	–	2	1	1	2	6
Brazil	119	111	97	113	93	533
Chile	34	7	10	13	15	79
Colombia	–	10	18	3	10	41
Costa Rica	–	1	2	1	–	4
Cuba	2	2	17	28	–	49
Dominican Republic	–	–	–	6	6	12
Ecuador	–	1	1	2	7	11
El Salvador	–	2	1	1	1	5
Guatemala	–	1	–	3	1	5
Haiti	–	1	–	–	–	1
Honduras	–	–	1	6	1	8
Jamaica	2	–	–	–	–	2
Mexico	75	45	132	150	55	457
Nicaragua	–	2	–	–	2	4
Panama	2	–	2	1	1	6
Paraguay	–	–	1	1	1	3
Peru	36	8	12	6	6	68
Suriname	–	–	1	–	–	1
Trinidad and Tobago	–	2	–	1	1	4
Uruguay	1	2	–	1	2	6
Venezuela	9	10	21	22	20	82
Total	302	222	333	389	241	1487

Sources: ICOLD, 1989; World Resources Institute, 1987.
[a] Completed or under construction.

irrigated land were added; by 1975 more than 90 000 ha were under irrigation. The Quinquennial Programme of Hydraulic Resources for 1976–1980 considered the possibility of reaching a total of 246 916 ha of cultivated land under irrigation by the end of the decade.

Dams in Asia and the Western Pacific

Asia's remarkable achievements in dam construction are led by China and India. With a population of over 1000 million people, China had 18 800 dams by 1986, compared with 17 400 in the rest of the world. India, with a population of 786 million in 1987, added 206 large dams in the 1980s. During the same period 21 were constructed in Indonesia (173 million people), and 22 in Malaysia (16 million) (Table 6). Thailand, with 53 million people, probably has the highest density of dams, having constructed 109 since 1961, 17 of them during the 1970s and 83 in the last ten years (ICOLD, 1989).

17

Table 6. Number of dams over 10 m high built in Asia (excluding Japan)

Country	Before 1961	1961–80	After 1980[a]
Afghanistan	2	–	–
Bangladesh	–	1	–
Cambodia	–	1	1
China[b]	337	875	321
Cyprus	5	27	16
Democratic People's Republic of Korea	34	27	9
India[b]	232	143	206
Indonesia	15	16	21
Iran (Islamic Republic of)	1	17	10
Iraq	1	4	8
Jordan	–	4	1
Lao People's Democratic Republic	–	1	–
Lebanon	2	3	–
Malaysia	4	12	22
Myanmar	–	1	3
Nepal	–	–	3
Pakistan	4	30	4
Philippines	4	3	6
Republic of Korea	257	368	140
Saudi Arabia	2	16	20
Singapore	–	2	1
Sri Lanka	44	25	10
Syrian Arab Republic	1	11	–
Thailand	–	29	80
Turkey	13	55	101
Viet Nam	–	1	–
Total	958	1672	983

Source: ICOLD, 1989.
[a] Completed or under construction.
[b] Over 30 m high.

The construction of dams has not been deferred by civil war or disturbance in certain Asian countries. Cambodia and the Lao People's Democractic Republic constructed large dams at Kirirom (1968) and Nam Ngum (1972), respectively. Myanmar completed two large dams at Mboye (1971) and Kinda (1986) and is now constructing two more, Sedawgyi I and II. Information is not easily accessible on some projects, such as hydroelectric developments in Sabah and Sarawak, which are not listed by the International Commission on Large Dams but are of ecological significance.

Agricultural irrigation systems

The pressure of population increase in the developing world clearly demands an expansion of agricultural production, the achievement of which requires intensification of water impoundment and irrigation. Changes in land utilization and distribution of irrigated land are shown in Table 7. In Africa, where the population may double in the next 25 years, only 30% of the land is suitable for food crops dependent on rainfall, and there are significant regional differences. Given the food demands for the world's increasing population it appears inevitable that more land will be irrigated. Houston (1977) suggested that 23 million ha of irrigated land would be needed in addition to the existing 50 million ha, including irrigated areas that required improvement or rehabilitation.

Irrigated agriculture contributes significantly to the world's food supply. Rice is the main food of 60% of the world's population, and is grown on 35% of the irrigated land (Coosemans & Mouchet, 1990). India has only a tenth as much surface area as Africa yet irrigates five times as much land. Only a twentieth of the cropped area in Africa is irrigated; in Egypt 98.6% of cropped land is irrigated; 70% of irrigated land in Africa is in four countries: Egypt, Madagascar, Nigeria and Sudan (FAO, 1987b). Since 1965, per capita agricultural production in Asia has increased at an average rate of 1.3%

Table 7. Utilization and irrigation of land

	Land area (thousands of hectares)				
	1965	**1973**	**1978**	**1983**	**1988**
Total land area	13 073 846	13 066 586	13 069 403	13 069 332	13 069 253
Area of arable and permanent crops	1 370 712	1 417 997	1 444 660	1 461 190	1 475 426
Area of irrigated land					
World	150 549	181 583	205 996	219 094	228 672
Africa	8 241	9 222	9 743	10 428	11 146
North and Central America	19 534	22 199	27 359	27 002	25 809
South America	5 047	6 244	7 131	7 961	8 755
Asia	96 924	117 280	129 524	137 299	142 757
Europe	9 535	12 286	13 993	15 389	17 297
Percentage of cropland irrigated (world)	10.98	12.81	14.26	14.99	15.5

Source: FAO (1989).

Table 8. Multipurpose and irrigation dams in south-east Asia

Name	Location	Type[a]	Power (MkWh/year)	Total cost (millions of US$)	Reservoir area (km²)	Irrigation Completion date	Irrigation Area (ha)
Indonesia							
Jatiluhur	Central Java	M	700	220	83	1967	260 000
Wonogiri	Central Java	M	28	262	80	–	23 200
Malaysia							
Kenyir	Trengganu State	M	1600	106	370	–	198 000
Muda/Pedu	Kedah	I	–	173	90	1970	105 200
Philippines							
Pantabangan	Central Luzon	M	32	123	853	1974	83 700

Thailand

Bhumiphol	Tak Province, Northern Region	M	1600	125	315	1964	404 600
Ubol Ratana	Khon Kaen Province, North-east Region	M	65	48	414	1966	48 000
Srinagarind	Kanchanaburi Province, Central Region	M	1271	221	419	1981	233 100
Lam Ta-kong	Nakhon-ratcha-sima Province, North-east Region	I	–	12	25	1969	38 527

a M: multipurpose; I: irrigation.
Source: Sornmani & Harinasuta, 1988.

per year, largely as a result of irrigation schemes. During the same period in Latin America, there has been little change, while in Africa there has been a decline of 1.4% per year (FAO, 1990). This contrasts with an increase in all regions of the total irrigated land in the same period.

By 1984, responding to food demand, 18 African and Latin American countries were irrigating 25 320 000 ha; the rate of expansion in Madagascar, Mali and Nigeria, exceeded 100% in the decade 1974–84.

Vast irrigable lands have been developed in Indonesia, Malaysia, the Phillippines and Thailand (Table 8). Thailand's Bhumiphol project covers 404 600 ha and at Srinagarind there are 233 100 ha. Jatiluhur in Central Java irrigates 260 000 ha, while Kenyir and Muda/Pedu irrigate 198 000 and 105 000 ha respectively. Seven of the nine projects listed in Table 8 also generate power.

In the São Francisco Valley of Brazil, 166 830 ha were irrigated in 1988 and it is anticipated that there will be 335 850 ha of irrigated land by 1993, a twofold increase in five years (CODEVASF, 1989).

A useful classification of countries has been devised in terms of the proportion of arable land under irrigation (Alexandratos, 1988). In most of the countries where over 30% of the arable land is under irrigation, namely Cuba, Egypt, Guyana, Islamic Republic of Iran, Iraq, Pakistan, Peru, Saudi Arabia, Suriname, and Yemen, there are major problems of one or more parasitic diseases including malaria, filariasis and schistosomiasis; the Republic of Korea and the Democratic People's Republic of Korea provide exceptions to this state of affairs.

At the country level there are three categories of irrigation system according to size:

- *Large plots (more than 500 ha).* These are usually state-financed, if not nationalized. They may be managed directly by the state or through a parastatal agency. Most systems are surface gravity-fed or pumped. The largest is the Gezira and its extensions in the Sudan. Others of comparable dimensions exist in Cameroon (Corporation for the Expansion and Modernization of Rice Cultivation in Yagoua) (SEMRY), Mali (Office de Niger), Zimbabwe (Hippo Estates), and elsewhere.

- *Medium plots (between 50 and 500 ha).* Their financing and management may be nationalized, cooperative or private; mostly surface irrigation is used. Examples are found in Madagascar (Mangoaky), Mauritania, and Niger (Tillaberry).

- *Small plots (less than 50 ha).* These are the most varied, including high- and low-water developments on flood plains, internal valleys and coastal swamps, lake shores, and systems involving small earth dams and gravity-fed manual and mechanical pumping methods from watercourses and wells. Independent smallholders or peasant groups have plots of this size, with only partial water control or dependence on high water levels. There are many examples in Ghana, Guinea, Kenya, Liberia, Mali, Senegal, and the United Republic of Tanzania.

The influence of the choice of an irrigation system (large or small scale, new or rehabilitated) on the dynamics of poverty are widely recognized. The tendency towards smaller-scale irrigation, using swamp management, river diversion or tubewells, should promote the participation of small producers in the economy (Fouya, 1990).

The potential for new irrigation developments in Chad, Egypt, Libyan Arab Jamahiriya, and Sudan is limited by the availability of water resources. The types of terrain, the limited number of large rivers, and the small alluvial valleys suggest that African irrigation will develop in small dispersed units. Planning experience in this area is limited (FAO, 1990). African countries in the subhumid zone, such as Ethiopia, Ghana, and the United Republic of Tanzania are now encouraging this scale of irrigation. The 1 300 000 ha of irrigated land in the West African countries of Benin, Burkina Faso, Chad, Côte d'Ivoire, Ghana, Mali, Mauritania, Niger, Nigeria (which has 850 000 ha), Senegal, and Togo, mostly in medium plots, represent 28% of the irrigable potential. However, in Burkina Faso only 14 000 ha of the potential 160 000 ha are actually irrigated. In the Mahgreb countries of Algeria, Libyan Arab Jamahiriya, Morocco, and Tunisia, there are more farmer-managed irrigated plots than in the rest of Africa except Madagascar and Nigeria.

Each year in the late 1970s and early 1980s some 5000 ha of Sahelian land were irrigated for the first time, but an equal area was lost due to waterlogging and salination. The delta of the Senegal River was the principal dry-season grazing area for migrant cattle herds in southern Mauritania and northern Senegal. After a river embankment was constructed the soil salinity became too high for economically sound agriculture and the southern part of the delta became a virtual desert (Drijvers, 1990).

Fisheries and aquaculture

Freshwater fish production increased from 7.6 to 10.1 million tonnes between 1980 and 1985. Freshwater aquaculture currently contributes about a third of this total and 10% of all managed fish production. As fish prices continue to rise it is expected that freshwater aquaculture will expand at an annual rate of 5.5%, doubling by the end of the century.

Rural aquaculture in Africa is a comparatively recent development, closely associated with agricultural communities and irrigation. It is a growing secondary economic activity although at present it accounts for only 1% of global aquaculture production. Women have a notable role in developing its potential (FAO/SIDA, 1990). In Zambia, 30–40% of rural households are headed by women and aquaculture offers a stable income as well as a food source.

Culture-based fishery development is considered feasible in almost any artificial water resource (Haight, 1990). Many programmes are promoting aquaculture in small bodies of water, which are ideal for fish production since they are shallow and may produce up to 1000 kg/ha per year because of their nutrient-rich run-off. Aquaculture for Local Community Development (ALCOM) is an interregional programme of FAO involving the countries of the Southern Africa Development Commercial Community: Angola, Botswana, Lesotho, Malawi, Mozambique, Namibia, Swaziland, United Republic of Tanzania, Zambia, and Zimbabwe. West Africa has a programme called Integrated Development of Artisanal Fisheries, and the Bay of Bengal Programme includes Bangladesh, India, Indonesia, Malaysia, Maldives, Sri Lanka, and Thailand.

In the basins of the São Francisco, Paraná and Uruguay Rivers in South America, the construction of high dams has reduced the reproductive potential of migratory fish. These are in high demand and their usual high prices mean that there has been a significant economic loss as well as a diminished protein intake for the local populations.

In an attempt to compensate for the negative economic and nutritional impact of dam construction, some hydroelectric enterprises are promoting ichthyological studies and aquaculture to adapt fish, some from Amazonia, to the new environment. Aquaculture is not without risk in these areas. The numerous artificial ponds in proximity to reservoirs are excellent habitats for snails (especially *Biomphalaria* spp.) and mosquitos. Drainage during cleaning operations and overflow during the rainy season can result in snails passing into the reservoirs. Different species of snail have been introduced into new areas through the transportation of fish, as with *Bulinus truncatus* in Jordan (Rey, 1979) or *Biomphalaria straminea,* of South American origin, into Hong Kong and China (Meier-Brook, 1974; Walker, 1978).

3.

Adverse health effects of water development schemes

Filariasis, malaria, onchocerciasis and schistosomiasis are the major parasitic diseases associated with the ecological and social changes in and around water resources projects (Table 9).

The most significant reported increases in disease prevalence and public health importance attributable to water development schemes concern schistosomiasis. Although this disease is not associated with mortality, as is malaria, or with the dramatic morbidity of elephantiasis due to lymphatic filariasis, in affected communities it is always recognized as a major health problem to which people attribute much of their misery. While this may not be documented in health statistics, since schistosomiasis is rarely a reportable disease (Iarotski & Davis, 1981), its frequency and severity in these schemes have been recorded.

The changes introduced by dam construction and other water resources projects create or aggravate health risks in different ways. With regard to parasitic diseases, the first effects are observed as a result of displacement, migration, settlement and employment. Since none of the parasitic diseases in question have major animal reservoirs, an infected person may be the first indication of risk.

Demographic and socioeconomic factors

One of the keys to health intervention in water resources projects is an understanding of human population dynamics. From the labour force to the peripheral settlements, the movements of people and vectors determine the extent and severity of adverse effects on health. The scale of these movements is enormous: in 1981, more than 600 000 Indian workers were present in the countries of the Eastern Mediterranean alone (Gunatilleke, 1985). Migratory movements, population resettlement and working conditions created by water resources projects are also sources of risk, these ones being linked more closely to human living conditions. In an

25

Table 9. Global distribution of major parasitic diseases associated with water resources development

	Number of endemic countries	Exposed population (millions)	Infected population (millions)
Schistosomiasis	74	600	200
Lymphatic filariasis	69	752	75
Onchocerciasis	34	166	25
Malaria	99	2200	275[a]

[a] In Africa alone.

Source: WHO Division of Control of Tropical Diseases.

interactive manner these movements are caused by and create vulnerability to disease in specific groups of people (Hammad & Mulholland, 1989).

Communities in the vicinity of large irrigation systems may have high illiteracy rates and poverty factors that have important health consequences. In the Sudan the situation has been aggravated by drought and famine, with increased frequency of diarrhoeal diseases, malaria and schistosomiasis (Taha & Merghani, 1990).

An increase in the density of human populations and the invasion of sylvatic ecosystems exacerbates the transmission of parasitic diseases. Other diseases are attributable to poor living conditions in settler communities. Overcrowding is responsible for a high incidence of respiratory infections and a relatively high prevalence of tuberculosis. The scarcity of domestic water and the absence of sanitary facilities in residential areas around dam-building sites lead to hyperendemicity of enteritis and other diarrhoeal diseases, as well as one of their important consequences, dehydration. In Latin America, houses constructed of dried mud are invaded and colonized by the triatomid vectors of Chagas disease.

On construction sites the arrival of large numbers of immigrants causes housing problems, increases in rent and food costs, unstable employment and unemployment.All these factors contribute to a lowering of nutritional status and a consequent increase in susceptibility to infection. A predominance of single men in the labour force promotes prostitution and leads to a high incidence of sexually transmitted diseases, particularly gonorrhoea and syphilis.

Such risks would have produced even more dramatic results in dam construction areas but for preventive health services and control measures. Sometimes the cost of control operations has been supported by project administrations. Such direct financial support has been particularly im-

Table 10. Influence of the Trans-Amazonian Highway on malaria prevalence in various states of Brazil

State	Prevalence of malaria (%)	
	Area of Trans-Amazonian Highway	Other areas
Maranhão	12.3	5.0
Para	14.5	3.9
Amazonas	17.7	7.4
Acre	22.8	1.9

Source: Ministry of Health, Brazil, 1976.

portant when risks were not foreseen or were not reduced by preventive measures.

A true appreciation of the influence of water resources projects on health risks requires specific surveys to collect pre- and post-impoundment data, with statistical analysis of disease rates within and outside the project zones. An example can be found in a study on the influence of the Trans-Amazonian Highway on the prevalence of malaria (Table 10; SUCAM, 1976).

Large dams are usually constructed in remote areas where the local population is comprised of poor peasants and fishermen. Modern construction enterprises displace people from reservoir sites and they are relocated by force or chance in nearby settlements. These movements disrupt their bonds with the environment with which they are familiar. Cultural traditions and a lack of technical orientation and basic education make it difficult for local people to enter the permanent labour force. Moreover, the lack of appropriate training programmes limits them to temporary work in deforestation or other manual labour. These people thus become marginalized in the local setting or they may migrate to other remote areas with an environment similar to that of their place of origin. In either case there are significant health risks for this vulnerable group.

Labour forces on dam construction sites come almost exclusively from distant areas. A significant proportion of the workers are permanent migrants, moving from one site to another. Technical and administrative staff are accommodated in residential enclaves with adequate basic services. On the other hand, the labourers and their families reside in surrounding slums. This unstable population may reach hundreds of thousands at the peak of construction.

In general, health risks are greatest in areas of high endemicity of disease with economically weak populations. Organizational and budgetary resources for appraisal of future risks and of needs for early preventive interventions are not usually available in projects of medium or small capacity. In countries or regions without adequate infrastructures for disease control, new projects may harm local populations and later require more costly procedures to cope with the situation.

Aggravation of health risks by ecosystem changes

Alterations in aquatic ecosystems directly modify the habitats, breeding patterns and, ultimately, the distribution and density of intermediate snail hosts and insect vectors. However, a water resources project does more than alter the distribution and flow of water. Deforestation, land occupation, soil degradation, and desertification may all contribute to ecosystem changes.

The intermediate snail hosts of schistosomiasis have preferential habitats (Chu et al., 1968; Hubendick, 1958; Watson, 1958). In Central and East Africa, irrigation systems tend to be populated predominantly by *Bulinus* species. The acidity of certain impoundments, reflecting the extent of inundated forest, inhibits the intermediate snail hosts of schistosomes.

Significant snail populations have been observed in the early stages of large water impoundments when vegetation is absent. Under these conditions, snails have been detected under rocks along the edges of the lakes. In the early stages of water impoundment, an overgrowth of floating or submerged vegetation consisting of *Pistia, Salvinia* and *Ceratophyllum* is an ideal snail habitat.

Man-made lakes differ from natural ones in their seasonal fluctuations in water level. The levels of natural lakes tend to vary more and are at their lowest in the winter, whereas artificial lakes are either stable or tend to be highest in the winter. These fluctuations have been dramatic in Lake Volta in recent years, when drought in northern Ghana was responsible for lowering the level of the lake by some 50 m. The isolation and exposure of *Bulinus* on the shore almost completely eliminated transmission.

Rodents and other mammals are important in the epidemiology of parasitic diseases. Over 30 domestic and wild mammals have been reported to be infected with *S. japonicum*. Most of these species participate in the ecosystems of water resources projects. Reports from Brazil, Kenya, and Senegal suggest that rodent populations in irrigation systems and water resources schemes can maintain the life cycle of *S. mansoni*, and that people entering the environment are at high risk of infection. This appears to be especially so in irrigated sugar cane fields; it is less so in rice fields.

In the Nile Delta the transmission of schistosomiasis in the irrigated zone is greatest in rice irrigation in the lowest land areas with the highest water usage. Wheat and vegetable cultivation tends to be on higher ground with limited water requirements and is associated with lower prevalence of schistosomiasis.The areas of mixed cultivation have intermediate prevalence. It has been suggested that increased salinity and the change from seasonal flooding to perennial irrigation after the completion of the Aswan High Dam led to the predominance of *Biomphalaria* over *Bulinus* in the Nile Delta (Abdel-Wahab et al., 1979).

Aquatic weeds tend to decrease the speed of water flow within irrigation systems. In the Sudan, canal banks tend to become overgrown with *Pancium repens, Cyperus rotundus* and *Ipomoea repens,* or with free-floating or anchored weeds such as *Potamogeton* spp., *Chara globulans, Najas* spp., and *Ottelia* spp. The introduction of herbivorous fish including the Chinese carp (*Ctenopharyngodon idella*) and *Tilapia zillii* and of fish that eat snails or mosquito larvae changes the ecosystem even further (Coates & Redding-Coates, 1981).

Odei (1973) studied the potential of aquatic plants to enhance snail habitats in Lake Volta. *Ceratophyllum,* a non-rooted submerged plant, is the favoured habitat of *Bulinus* (Klumpp & Chu, 1977). Among the free-floating plants, *Salvinia, Pistia* and *Spirodela,* the latter contributes to the spread of snails. Aquatic plants at the lake margin, such as *Polygonum, Vossia, Alternanthera* and *Jussiaea,* tend to survive flooding and contribute to sudd formation and the establishment of snail habitats.

The modifications of ecology that influence mosquito breeding and population density begin with deforestation or the inundation of forest or savanna areas. Such changes favour *Anopheles gambiae,* which is attracted to sunlight and is the main vector of malaria in Africa. Its potential breeding sites and population density increase with environmental degradation.

In the Amazon region of Brazil there is a direct correlation between the proximity of human settlements to the forest fringe and the transmission of malaria by *Anopheles darlingi* at large dam construction sites. In south-east Asia, however, forest clearing for water resources development militates against *Anopheles dirus,* which is heliophobic.

It has been suggested that, in addition to the negative effect of the reduction of water speed in *Simulium* breeding sites, overgrowth of water hyacinth (*Eichhornia crassipes*), imported from the Americas into Africa, consumes essential nutrient elements.

At impoundment sites in Africa, *Anopheles gambiae* and *A. funestus* can be anticipated; in Turkey *A. sacharovi* predominates. In Asian artificial lakes with heavy vegetation, particularly *Pistia* and *Salvinia, Mansonia* mosquitos proliferate and are important vectors of lymphatic filariasis caused by *Brugia malayi*.

Agricultural irrigation systems provide the greatest potential for increased populations of arthropod and snail vectors of parasitic diseases (Bradley, 1977; Brunet-Jailly, 1982; FAO, 1987a; IRRI, 1988; White, 1978). In irrigation systems the heliotropic species are at peak densities in the early stages of the rice-growing season: the *Anopheles gambiae* complex, *A. arabiensis* in Africa, *A. culicifacies* in India, and *A. sinensis* in China. However, as the rice reaches a height at which sufficient shadow is provided, *A. funestus*, a potent vector of malaria in Africa, may predominate. The *A. gambiae* complex proliferates extensively in artificial bodies of water, whereas *A. funestus* produces stable populations in shaded water. On the plains of India, malaria epidemics are associated with *A. culicifacies* after heavy monsoon rains and subsequent flooding or waterlogging in poorly managed irrigation systems. In China, *A. sinensis* breeds well in overgrown drainage canals or storage tanks in irrigation systems.

Near Bobo-Dioulasso in Burkina Faso the density of *A. gambiae* in the rice irrigation systems is ten times that in the surrounding savanna. Paradoxically, the sporozoite rate among mosquitos is ten times lower, and consequently the expected increase in malaria transmission has not occurred (Robert et al., 1985).

In the rice agro-ecosystem in Mandla District, Madhya Pradesh, India, the density of *Anopheles* breeding sites is inversely proportional to the distance from the villages. *A. culicifacies* breeds in rice fields where the plants are up to 20 cm high. Where they are taller, shading allows *A. theobaldi* and *A. splendidus* to predominate. *A. fluviatilis* breeds in the drainage irrigation canals throughout the rice-growing season. Breeding sites generally increase in number following the rains (Singh et al., 1989).

In the Mahaweli project area in Sri Lanka, the ecological changes at various stages of development influenced the malaria pattern. After construction, pools formed in the river bed below the dam and breeding sites were thus created for *A. culicifacies*, the main vector of *Plasmodium vivax*. Malaria epidemics occurred nearby and control was achieved by periodically releasing water and flushing the river bed. Borrow pits and temporary wells created breeding sites for *A. culicifacies* and *A. subpictus*. Deforestation reduced the animal populations on which feeding usually took place, and so the overcrowded settlements of temporary shelters became sites of malaria epidemics. The subsequent poor maintenance and drainage of the vast irrigation system increased the potential for transmission throughout the year (P. Herath, personal communication, 1990).

African Region

The major river basins of Africa are being subjected to enormous environmental modifications as a result of water resources development. The West African river basins provide numerous examples of the health impact of water resources development (Brown & Wright, 1985).

Burkina Faso

In Burkina Faso a rice irrigation scheme in the valley of the Tiao River was started in 1955 and soon became an intense area of onchocerciasis transmission (Le Berre, 1971). Endemicity was initially low, yet virtually the entire population was affected by 1962. Eye lesions were observed in children aged 10–14 years, and 50% of people aged over 40 were blind. Engineering modifications of the spillways were relatively unsuccessful for vector control (Quélennec et al., 1968). Degradation of the rice fields was subsequently associated with a decrease in prevalence.

In south-west Burkina Faso a high prevalence of *Wuchereria bancrofti* infection (40%) and clinical signs of hydrocele or elephantiasis were noted in Tinguela, where the growing of irrigated crops was the main agricultural activity (Brengues, 1975). Schistosomiasis is widespread in all irrigation systems (LeBras et al., 1982) and hydroelectric dam reservoirs (Bani et al., 1990).

Burundi

In 1950 a land reclamation and irrigation scheme was begun in the Rusizi valley, and led to the migration of over 50 000 people from the highlands. By the time the malaria and schistosomiasis control programme was established in 1966 (Mission d'Assainissement de la Plaine de la Rusizi), the number of cases of schistosomiasis had increased 30-fold (Gryseels, 1990).

Cameroon

In addition to some medium-size dams, many small ones have been built in the Mandara Mountains in northern Cameroon during the past 15

31

years (Ripert et al., 1979; Ripert, 1984). Small dams in towns are mainly to provide drainage for land reclamation, but over 100 small artificial lakes are used for fish culture. Some of the earthworks provide water for rice-growing. These developments have led to a considerable increase in the prevalence of schistosomiasis, onchocerciasis, and malaria (Roche et al., 1987). Furthermore, the lack of an adequate water supply for the people in this area caused an increase in dracunculiasis (guinea–worm disease).

Cameroon's Department of Mayo Danai is the location of a major rice-producing scheme conducted by the Corporation for the Expansion and Modernization of Rice Cultivation in Yagoua (SEMRY). The first two phases of this project, SEMRY I and SEMRY II, have brought 19 000 ha under irrigation. In its first stage, SEMRY III is developing an additional area of 600 ha for irrigation.

In this area the prevalence of urinary schistosomiasis was estimated to be about 15% in the 1950s; in the early 1960s its prevalence among schoolchildren was about 30%, and by the late 1960s the prevalence rate was about 40%. It remained at least at this level in all subsequent surveys (Mott et al., 1986). The mean prevalence in nine villages with about 12 000 residents around Yagoua in SEMRY I in 1982 was 43.1%. For direct employees of the enterprise the corresponding figure was 14.3% (Jannin et al., 1982). In SEMRY II between 1979 and 1985 the overall prevalences in different villages ranged from zero to 61% (Audibert, 1982; Audibert et al., 1983, 1990). Allowing for migration over this period, however, the prevalence of malaria and schistosomiasis remained stable. Within this area, Audibert (1986) estimated that a 10% increase in the prevalence of schistosomiasis resulted in a 4.9% decrease in rice output.

The Lagdo Dam was built in 1982 on the Benoue river, creating a reservoir of more than 500 km^2. Attracted by the irrigated agriculture and fishing potential, large numbers of people migrated from elsewhere in Cameroon as well as from Chad and Nigeria. The prevalence of urinary schistosomiasis in the area in 1968 was about 15% (Doumenge et al., 1987) and S. mansoni was reported around the provincial capital in Garoua, downstream from the dam. In 1986, the prevalence of urinary schistosomiasis in 15 fishing villages reached 43% and S. mansoni infection was up to 36% in the same villages (Robert et al., 1989).

Côte d'Ivoire

The dam across the Bandama Valley, impounding Lake Kossou, was completed in 1972. The prevalence of S. haematobium infection before impoundment ranged from 5% to 42% (Deschiens & Cornu, 1976). A marked rise in urinary and intestinal schistosomiasis is expected in this area, but there are no recent published data. However, *Bulinus globosus*, *Bu. truncatus rohlfsi*, *Bu. forskalii* and *Biomphalaria pfeifferi* are widespread. As with other large impoundments, such as that of Lake Volta in Ghana, onchocerciasis increased downstream from the dam and decreased in the lake bed and upstream.

In the last ten years, two more large dams have been completed: the Buyo Dam on the Sassandra River in the forest zone of western Côte d'Ivoire and the Taabo Dam on the Bandama River in a deforested area below Lake Kossou. In 1982 both *S. haematobium* and *S. mansoni* were detected in local children and in a third of migrants. Within two years of the completion of both dams, populations of *Bulinus*, particularly *Bu. forskalii*, and of *Biomphalaria pfeifferi*, had increased relative to pre-impoundment levels (Sellin & Simonkovitch, 1983).

Focal transmission of schistosomiasis in small agricultural reservoirs in central Côte d'Ivoire is increasing (N'Goran, 1987), but no comprehensive information on the overall situation in Côte d'Ivoire is available.

Ethiopia

In the Wonji-Shewa Sugar Estate the prevalence of *S. mansoni* was less than 0.5% from its opening in 1954 until 1964 but by 1984 it had reached 19.4% (Tedla et al., 1989). In the Melka Sadi irrigation scheme, which began in 1972, *Bi. pfeifferi* was first identified within a year and after three years it was well established throughout the canal system.

Schistosomiasis due to *S. mansoni* is endemic along the upper reaches of the Awash valley, particularly on irrigated farms. The prevalence among migrant labourers ranges from 0.8% to 15.2% although the disease is not endemic in their areas of origin. The prevalence among schoolchildren, including the offspring of migrants, reaches 72% in some schools. In contrast the rate of urinary schistosomiasis is less than 2% among all migrant farm populations except in one area where local transmission is high (Kloos & Lemma, 1977; Haile-Meskal & Kloos, 1989).

S. haematobium infection was first recognized in two people from Gewane in the Middle Awash Valley in 1956. During the 1970s, irrigation schemes were promoted throughout the Gewane flood plain and the risk of schistosomiasis was identified (Haile-Meskal et al., 1985). A survey in one village in the midst of these developments found the prevalence of urinary schistosomiasis to be 54%.

The Water Resources Development Authority of the Ethiopian Resources Commission is undertaking a flood-control and irrigation project in the Gumara and Ribb flood plains on the shores of Lake Tana in Debre Tabor and Libo provinces, Gondar Region; 12 000 hectares will eventually be irrigated. The mean prevalence of *S. mansoni* infection in 11 surveyed sites within the project area was only 1.6%, while the prevalence in three surrounding communities was as high as 34% in schoolchildren (Lo et al., 1989). More alarming was the earlier recognition, in another settlement near Lake Tana, that the incidence of *S. mansoni* infection among new arrivals was 527 per 1000 persons in a 4-month period (Ayele & Tiruneh, 1982).

The Middle Beles irrigation project located south-west of Lake Tana and funded jointly by the Governments of Ethiopia and Italy was expected to cover over 65 000 hectares of alluvial plain by completion in 1989. In 1986, a survey of school-age children in 29 localities in the project area showed that up to 68% of those aged 10-14 years were infected with *S. mansoni* and the prevalence of malaria was 2% (Teklehaimanot & Fletcher, 1990).

Ghana

Lake Volta, the largest artificial impoundment, was created by the completion of a dam across the Volta River at Akosombo in 1964. By 1969 it was over 500 km long; its shoreline is over 5000 km in length and its surface area of 8500 km² is about 3% of that of the country.

Extensive surveys in 1955 by the Ministry of Health indicated a relatively high prevalence of urinary schistosomiasis (*S. haematobium*) around the lower reaches of the Volta River and low prevalence (5–10%) in the Volta Basin above Akosombo, in the area that was later to be impounded. As early as 1969 the prevalence of *S. haematobium* infection among children in lakeside communities was about 90%. The adverse effects of Lake Volta in this respect were indicated by the low prevalence of the disease in hinterland communities along a 7-km transect from the lake, associated with a decreasing dependence on the lake for domestic water needs (UNDP/WHO, 1979). *S. mansoni* has not been recorded in Lake Volta itself.

Along the lower Volta, downstream from the Akosombo Dam, the rapids at Senchi and Kpong provided breeding sites for *Simulium* in the 1970s, resulting in onchocerciasis prevalence of 40–50% in the area (Volta River Authority, 1977). These breeding sites were destroyed when the area was flooded on the construction of the Kpong Dam in 1981.

The Kpong Dam, some 25 km below the Akosombo Dam, resulted in the creation of a small lake of some 3500 ha, which immediately became infested with submerged and floating aquatic plants, including *Ceratophyllum* and *Pistia*, and with the bottom-rooted plants *Potamogeton* and *Vallisneria*. Intermediate snail hosts of *Schistosoma*, namely *Bu. globosus*, *Bu. truncatus* and *Biomphalaria pfeifferi*, are now found in the lake. Prevalence rates of 55% for *S. haematobium* and 35% for *S. mansoni* have been recorded in the population in this area.

Both urinary and intestinal schistosomiasis are prevalent in the area from Kpong to Ada in the Volta estuary (Odei, 1973). Prevalence rates of 7–52% for *S. mansoni* (Wen & Chu, 1984) and 88% for *S. haematobium* have been recorded among riparian communities. It is noteworthy that, before the dams were built at Akosombo and Kpong, schistosomiasis in the lower Volta was predominantly urinary and confined to the flood plains of the Tongu area but was not found in the River Volta channel itself (Onori et al., 1963; Odei, 1977).

The ecological and social changes induced another change in parasitic disease patterns. In 1973 it was predicted that the lake itself would become an important navigation route by which people with sleeping sickness (African trypanosomiasis) would move from foci in northern Ghana to the forest areas of the south in proximity to the lake. Tsetse flies (*Glossina*) were widespread in the natural southern forests. Before 1973, no human disease had been reported but increased contact of people with flies was predicted (Kuzoe, 1973). This prediction has proved correct; since 1975 cases of trypanosomiasis have been reported throughout the south (Agadzi, 1986).

In the Upper Region of Ghana between 1951 and 1965, 185 small dams were built with support from the United States Agency for International Development. The prevalence of urinary schistosomiasis in the areas with these dams was 45.3%; that in areas with only traditional water supplies was 19.8% (Hunter, 1981). A similar pattern was observed in Ketu District among schoolchildren in 13 villages. The rate of urinary schistosomiasis was significantly higher (up to 54%) in villages where the small dam reservoirs were poorly maintained (Zijlmans et al., 1989).

All of Ghana's water conservation projects have become infested with *Bulinus* species (*Bu. globosus* and/or *Bu. truncatus*) and *S. haematobium* (Odei, 1981). These projects include: Vea and Tono Dams for irrigation in northern Ghana; Okyereko and Mankessim Dams for irrigation in the Central Region; Nwabi and Barekese Dams for water supply in the Ashanti Region; Kakum Dam for water supply in the Central Region; Dawyhenya and Ashiaman Dams for irrigation in the Greater Accra

Region; and Weija Dam for both water supply and irrigation in the Greater Accra Region.

The Barekese Reservoir was invaded by *Mansonia* and other mosquitos soon after its construction in the early 1970s. The Okyereko irrigation system is infested with mosquitos and malaria transmission is now intense in this rice-growing area.

At the Soe Dam, there was a marked increase in the prevalence of onchocerciasis due to the high water speed in the dam spillway 1.0–1.3 m/sec) and the spillway surface, which created ideal conditions for *Simulium* breeding (WHO Regional Office for Europe, 1983).

Kenya

The Taita-Taveta smallholder irrigation scheme, inaugurated in 1928, now covers more than 1000 ha. The current prevalence of schistosomiasis (both *S. mansoni* and *S. haematobium*) is about 70%.

The largest of the six irrigation schemes under the authority of the National Irrigation Board, the Mwea Irrigation Scheme, covering 5836 ha, was initiated in 1952 in the upper Tana River Basin in the foothills of Mount Kenya. A survey in 1956 indicated that schistosomiasis was not endemic. The first case was reported in 1959; reported prevalences increased from 12.5% in 1966 to 24.4% in 1971. In 1972, prevalences of up to almost 80% were reported in villages surrounding the scheme (Waiyaki, 1987).

The Ahero rice irrigation scheme (Kano I) was established in 1968 on 840 ha in the Kano plain of western Kenya. In 1971, prevalences of *S. haematobium* and *S. mansoni* infection among schoolchildren were 3.5% and 4.2% respectively. The distribution of both *Bulinus* and *Biomphalaria* was patchy in the area. A systematic programme of molluscicide application and treatment of infected persons has subsequently kept the prevalence around 1% (Waiyaki, 1987).

Malaria due to *P. falciparum* is endemic in the area of the irrigation schemes. The prevalences of malaria at Mwea and Hola are respectively 26% and 54% higher than in the nonirrigated surrounding areas (WHO/FAO/UNEP, 1990). The prevalence of malaria also increased in the Ahero, Kano and Mwea schemes in association with the ideal breeding sites for *Anopheles gambiae*. In the Mwea irrigation scheme, *Anopheles pharoensis* is now also an important vector (Mukiama & Mwangi, 1989). In the Pekerra irrigation scheme, malaria transmission is now established but schistosomiasis has not yet been reported (Ngindu, 1990).

Mosquito surveys in the irrigated and nonirrigated areas of the Kano Plain project, in Nyanza Province, show that in the former there has been a reduction in the number of species and a change in the composition of the mosquito population, with about a fourfold increase in the house-entry rate. Following the growth of settlement in the area, an increase in malaria transmission was to be expected (Surtees, 1970, 1975). In 1988 it was observed that the prevalence of malaria in this area was 19.3%.

In some parts of Kenya there have traditionally been widespread earth excavations at the base of low slopes to retain surface water. These are commonly known as "hifir dams". In other areas the damming of ground seepage makes it possible to have rice fields or garden plots (Highton, 1974). According to Sturrock (personal communication, 1989), there was an extensive programme of small dam construction in the 1950s and 1960s, especially in the Machakos area. Most of these dams have fallen into disuse because of either silting or breaching of the spillways. Of the few surviving dams, none have persistent populations of *Biomphalaria* although *Bulinus africanus*, transmitting bovine schistosomiasis, is some-times present.

The Hola irrigation scheme, a cotton, maize and groundnut cul-tivation project of 875 hectares, was established in the 1950s in the lower Tana River Basin. By 1965 the prevalence of schistosomiasis among Pokomo children of school age was 70%; and in 1982 the prevalence in Pokomo and Orma schoolchildren was 90% (Waiyaki, 1987). *S. haema-tobium* rates of 90% were found in five of nine primary schools in the cotton project area; and in a newly settled area in the Machakos district, in nine schools the mean *S. mansoni* rate was 84%, many children suffering from disease of the liver and spleen (Jordan, 1985).

In the Tana River Basin Hydroelectric Scheme, involving the re-servoirs of the Masinga, Kindarum, Gitaru, Kamburu and Kiambere Dams within a distance of 100 km, increased malaria rates, persistent leishmaniasis, and schistosomiasis transmission are reported. The possibil-ity has been raised that increased rodent populations have contributed to the transmission of schistosomiasis (Ngindu, 1990).

In the Baringo District of Rift Valley Province, *S. mansoni* infection in children has recently been reported for the first time, in associ-ation with small dams constructed for land reclamation (Muigai et al., 1989).

Liberia

The St Paul River Development Hydroelectric Power Scheme, com-pleted in 1982, has been associated with an increase in malaria and schis-tosomiasis (WHO Regional Office for Europe, 1983).

Madagascar

Schistosomiasis is highly endemic in all irrigation systems in Madagascar (Doumenge et al., 1987). The prevalence of urinary schistosomiasis in the Lower Mangoky Irrigation Scheme at the outset, between 1966 and 1971, was low (Degremont, 1973). In Tsaramandroso the rate of infection rose from 6.6% in 1968 to 60% in 1974 (Pasteur Institute of Madagascar, 1975). In an irrigation project in Ambilobe, the rate of infection with *S. haematobium* reached 60% in the peripheral villages (Breuil et al., 1983b). The prevalence of urinary schistosomiasis in two schools within an irrigation scheme in Ankilavo in western Madagascar was 69%, while outside the scheme the prevalence was 7% (Howarth et al., 1988).

Mali

One year before construction of the Sélingué Dam in 1980, urinary schistosomiasis was absent in four villages around the future reservoir area and the prevalence rate was less than 20% in six other villages in the area. Three years after impoundment, *S. haematobium* was present in every village. Prevalence exceeded 20% in eight villages, reaching over 40% in one of them. A wide variation in *S. mansoni* prevalence among villages was observed before and after impoundment (Brinkmann et al., 1988; Traore, 1988).

Table 11. *Prevalence of schistosomiasis by environmental zone in Mali*[a]

Zone	Prevalence of schistosomiasis (%)		Prevalence of heavy infections of schistosomiasis (%)	
	Urinary	**Intestinal**	**Urinary**	**Intestinal**
Large irrigated area (Office du Niger management)	64.4	53.9	15.9	24.5
Small dams (Bandiagara District)	67.2	12.0	27.9	1.4
Riverine communities (River Niger)	19.9	1.9	4.5	0.6
No water development (savanna villages)	13.4	1.6	2.2	0.3

[a] Excluding Sélingué.
Adapted from Brinkmann et al., 1988.

The prevalence of urinary and intestinal schistosomiasis (S. haematobium and S. mansoni) is highest in areas of irrigation: the Office du Niger zone, with its canals and rice fields, had rates of 64.4% and 53.9% respectively. Near small dams in the Bandiagara district the rates were 67.2% and 12.0% respectively. The prevalence rates were notably smaller in the zone of the Sélingué dam (31.8% and 4.4%) and even lower in communities along the River Niger (19.9% and 1.9%). The lowest prevalences (13.4% and 1.6% respectively) were observed in savanna villages without water resources development (Table 11). The rate of urinary schistosomiasis is five times greater in irrigated areas than in traditional villages, while the rate of severe infection (shown by many schistosome eggs in the urine) is seven times higher. The difference in risk of intestinal schistosomiasis is even greater: serious infection is virtually absent in the villages without irrigation but increases to about 25% where there is irrigation (Brinkmann et al., 1988).

Niger

The extensive irrigation schemes along the River Niger around Niamey are foci of intense transmission of S. haematobium (Malek, 1985; Sellin et al., 1983a, 1983b). In some areas all children of school age are infected. Moreover, up to 80% of infected children and over 60% of infected adults have disease of the genitourinary tract detectable by ultrasound (Lamothe et al., 1989).

Nigeria

Completion of the Kainji Dam in 1970 created a lake of 1600 km² with lakeside prevalence of S. haematobium of up to 62% in some villages. Prevalence and intensity were much higher around the lake than in nearby New Bussa (Dazo & Biles, 1972, 1973). On the opposite, eastern, side of Lake Kainji the prevalence of both urinary and intestinal schistosomiasis adjacent to an irrigation project was up to 30% (Adekolu-John, 1983; Adekolu-John & Abolarin, 1986). Onchocerciasis continues to be a major public health problem: the prevalence in 13 villages in 1985 was 28.5% (Edungbola et al., 1986).

In 1977, prior to the construction of the Jebba Dam (which was completed in 1982, creating a reservoir about 100 km long), it was predicted that onchocerciasis, trypanosomiasis, malaria and schistosomiasis would be important public health problems around this impoundment (Adekolu-John, 1980). No field assessment is yet available.

In the Funtua Agricultural Development Project of Malumfashi District, 16 earth dams were built and 64 more were planned for construction in the Ruwan Sanyi area. The overall prevalence of urinary schistosomiasis was 13.5%, the rate among 5–15-year-old boys being 41.2% in 1976 (Pugh & Gilles, 1978). At the Ruwan Sanyi Dam, snail habitats were almost completely destroyed during construction and filling, yet, within six months, dense populations of *Bulinus globosus* colonized the entire lake margin (Tayo & Jewsbury, 1978).

In Kano State, the Water Resources and Engineering Construction Agency has plans for construction of 37 major dams, half of which have been completed. In the Tomas and Rimin Gado dam areas the prevalence of urinary schistosomiasis has reached 37% (Betterton et al., 1988).

In the South Chad Irrigation Project, below Lake Chad in Borno State, the prevalence of urinary schistosomiasis was as high as 66% in some villages (Noamesi & Morcos, 1974) and the snail hosts are widespread (Betterton, 1984).

Senegal

A feasibility study by the United States Agency for International Development and the *Organisation pour la mise en valeur de la Vallée du Fleuve Sénégal* (OMVS) concluded that it was not possible to be sure how the planned irrigation in the Senegal River Basin would affect the prevalence of human schistosomiasis, but that there might be little or no increase. This boded well for the proposed further development of 24 000 ha for rice-growing on completion of the barrage (Miller, 1981). However, Vercruysse et al. (1985) published data that contradicted these conclusions. *Bulinus senegalensis* was established in the newly created rice fields, and, where this occurred along the Senegal River, for example at Lampsar and Guède Chantier, there was a concomitant increase in urinary schistosomiasis. Regular surveillance for new foci of *S. haematobium* in the rice fields was strongly advised. Furthermore, it had been argued that the two major water impoundment projects planned for the Senegal Valley, Diama at St Louis and Manantali at Bafoulabé (completed in 1988, displacing 12 000 persons and creating a 45 000 ha reservoir to irrigate 225 000 ha), would increase snail and mosquito populations and the risks of human disease (Malek & Chaine, 1989).

The first dam on the Senegal River was constructed at Taouey at Richard Toll in 1948. This stopped the seasonal flood from backflowing into Lake Guiers, permitting the irrigation of 6000 ha for rice cultivation and subsequently for sugar cane production.

The Diama Dam, a gate structure with an embankment on the Senegal River at St Louis, completed in August 1986, blocks saltwater intrusion during the dry season and has created a reservoir for irrigation and industrial installations. Surveillance by the laboratory of the health centre in Richard Toll began in May 1987. The first cases of *S. mansoni* infection were reported one and a half years after the dam became operational in early 1988. In the last quarter of 1989, 71.5% of 2086 routine stool examinations were positive (Talla et al., 1990). Increased populations of rodents (*Arvicanthus niloticus*, *Mastomys huberti* and *M. erythroleucus*) with focally high levels of infection in this area may significantly change the pattern of transmission (Duplantier et al., 1990).

Malaria was the most important public health problem in this area before the construction of the dam and the irrigation system. It remains a problem, and there are now also high rates of tick-borne borreliosis (Trape et al., 1991).

Sierra Leone

Over the past decade, agriculture in Sierra Leone has become increasingly geared for swamp rice cultivation. The Peace Corps, the World Bank and the European Community have supported this trend. *S. haematobium* and *S. mansoni* infections were observed in 95% and 50% respectively of 74 villages with a combined population of more than 25 000 (White et al., 1982).

In the Kono diamond belt the prevalence of *S. mansoni* was higher than that of *S. haematobium* in 1987 although it had not been reported in Blacklock's earlier surveys (Blacklock, 1924). In Yengama, the headquarters of the National Diamond Mining Corporation, the prevalence of both *S. haematobium* and *S. mansoni* was over 25% in 1989. The area of transmission of *S. mansoni* appears to be growing (White et al., 1989).

Swaziland

Between 1952 and 1954 the Department of Health reported that urinary schistosomiasis was already widely distributed and that *S. mansoni* had been found for the first time on irrigated estates of the low veld. On two estates between 1958 and 1964 the prevalence of *S. haematobium* ranged between 53% and 75% and that of *S. mansoni* from 21% to 70%. In 1977–78 it was reported that the prevalence of *S. mansoni* among field workers on three neighbouring estates ranged from 33.3% to 59.9% (Logan, 1983).

United Republic of Tanzania

At Ifakara in the Kilombero District of Morogoro Region, 49 bodies of water, most of them man-made, were surveyed and found to be infested with *Bulinus globosus* and/or *Bulinus nasutus*, and up to 71% of school-children were infected with *S. haematobium* (Zumstein, 1983).

In 1978 the potential for the spread of both urinary and intestinal schistosomiasis around the proposed Lake Mtera development was described (Matovu, 1978).

Zambia

The Zambezi River dam in the Kariba Gorge, completed in 1959, created Lake Kariba to provide hydroelectric power for neighbouring countries. It was the first of the large man-made lakes (Van Der Lingen, 1973). Before 1964, while the water was still rising, it seems that there was no transmission of schistosomiasis. Subsequently, the wealth of organic matter deriving from the decomposition of submerged vegetation provided a suitable environment for the spread of *Salvinia auriculata* which, in turn, proved favourable for the multiplication of snail vectors of *Schistosoma*. By 1968, the transmission of both intestinal and urinary schistosomiasis was intense in some areas (Hira, 1970).

The current status of schistosomiasis around Lake Kariba and in the Gwembe, Mpongwe and Kafue irrigation schemes is not known. However, the Ministry of Health maintains strict surveillance and control in the tourist areas alongside Lake Kariba.

In Zambia, *Biomphalaria* spp. and other snails are often abundant in seepages below the walls of small dams where people have their vegetable gardens, and there is a high risk of transmission at such sites (R.F. Sturrock, personal communication, 1989).

Zimbabwe

In 1968, before control measures were established in the agricultural Hippo Valley and Triangle Estates of the south-eastern low veld, the prevalence of both *S. haematobium* and *S. mansoni* had risen to above 55% among children of school and pre-school age (Evans, 1983).

Extensive national surveys reveal continuing strong associations between commercial irrigation and schistosomiasis (Taylor & Makura, 1985). On 115 commercial agricultural estates the prevalence of *S. haematobium* exceeded 20%, and on 43 of these estates the prevalence was above 60%. The prevalence of *S. mansoni* (intestinal) schistosomiasis was elevated by irrigation to more than 33% on 19 estates. On ten agricultural estates the two diseases coexisted at levels exceeding 20% for *S. mansoni* and 60% for *S. haematobium*.

Eastern Mediterranean Region

Egypt

Along the Nile Valley, high population densities together with intensive agricultural practices and frequent and prolonged contact with water have led to some of the most dramatic changes ever observed in the prevalence of schistosomiasis (Abdallah, 1978).

The construction of the Low Dam at Aswan in the early 1930s allowed perennial irrigation in a number of provinces. Between 1934 and 1937 in Kom Ombo, Upper Egypt, the conversion from traditional irrigation (yearly flooding, one crop) to perennial irrigation (year-round water, one or more crops) resulted in increases in the prevalence of urinary schistosomiasis from 0% to 34% in Sibaia, 7% to 50% in Kilh, 2% to 64% in Bemban, and 11% to 75% in Mansouria (Khalil Bey, 1949).

A malaria epidemic in Upper Egypt in 1942–43, which caused 130 000 deaths, followed an invasion of *Anopheles gambiae* from the Sudan (Farid, 1977), and must be seen as a consequence of water development.

The formation of Lake Nasser (6500 km^2) on the Nile at the Aswan High Dam, constructed between 1960 and 1968, caused considerable changes in the ecology of the region; 500 000 ha of unproductive land were reclaimed and the continuous irrigation was achieved of some 300 000 ha of land that formerly had been only intermittently irrigated. In other parts of the country it had already been found that the change from intermittent to permanent irrigation raised the prevalence of schistosomiasis from 0–5% to 60% and above.

In 1971, 61% of the fishermen who came to settle near Lake Nasser had schistosomiasis, whereas the rate among the former inhabitants of Abu Simbel was only 9%. The population density around the lake remains very low but the situation could worsen if settlement plans were implemented.

The Aswan High Dam also contributed to a sudden, unexpected increase in the transmission of intestinal schistosomiasis (*S. mansoni*), while there was a decrease in urinary schistosomiasis (*S. haematobium*) in the Nile Delta as well as in Upper Egypt (Schistosomiasis Symposium, 1979; Abdel-Wahab et al., 1979). The prevalence of *S. mansoni* is highest in governorates ·where rice production is intense. *Biomphalaria alexandrina*, the intermediate host of *S. mansoni* in Egypt, has spread southwards from the Nile Delta through the Aswan governorate (Mallet & Aboul-Ela, 1979). Although large-scale molluscicide application for snail control has been carried out in Middle and Upper Egypt since 1977, *B. alexandrina* is still present in some canals. In 1980, 30% of the fishermen on Lake Nasser were infected with *S. haematobium* and some cases of *S. mansoni* infection were also observed (Strickland, 1982). These observations signal a risk of possible spread and entrenchment of intestinal schistosomiasis from the Nile Delta to the Sudan border.

Jordan

In 1975 *Bulinus truncatus*, an intermediate host for *S. haematobium*, was discovered in a cement reservoir that fed periodically into a canal carrying water from the Yarmouk River to farms in the Jordan Valley. In 1978 the same host was found at Jerash within the watershed of the new King Talal Dam on the Zarqa river. Since 24% of labourers entering Jordan are estimated to be infected, there is clearly a risk of *in situ* transmission. In 1984–85 the first autochthonous cases of schistosomiasis were reported in Karak Governorate, at some distance from the above sites (WHO, 1987b). As yet transmission has not been confirmed in water resources projects (Saliba et al., 1986).

Oman

In 1982 it was observed that *Biomphalaria arabica* was present in Wad Arazat, the source of water for irrigation of the Royal Arazat Farm. About 7% of the local farm labourers were infected with *S. mansoni*. This was the first reported evidence of transmission of *S. mansoni* in Oman (Githaiga, 1983).

Saudi Arabia

In the Al Baha Region, 18 of 21 reservoirs created in recent years have become densely populated with both *Biomphalaria arabica* and *Bulinus truncatus*. Transmission of *S. mansoni* is now well established.

A large dam in the Najran Region, on the border of Yemen, became infested with *Bu. beccarii*, the main intermediate host of *S. haematobium* in Saudi Arabia, and with *Bi. arabica*. The prevalence of urinary schistosomiasis has subsequently increased downstream of the dam (Arfaa, 1988a).

Other changes include the recent infestation of a large reservoir near Madina City by *Bi. arabica*.

The construction of small dams for water retention has created breeding conditions suitable for the spread of mosquitos of the *Anopheles gambiae* complex and for malaria transmission.

Somalia

Throughout the Lower Shabelle Valley there are pump- and gravity-fed irrigation schemes for agricultural production. The prevalence of *S. haematobium* is above 90% among school-age children in some villages of this region, the situation having been exacerbated by low rates of school attendance and the employment of children in the fields (Hagi, 1986). Schistosomiasis has been reported in the Juba Valley and there is a risk of irrigation-promoted increases in transmission (Jobin, 1989).

Sudan

The Gezira irrigation system covers 850 000 ha and consists of the original Gezira scheme of 1925 and the Managil extension, finished in 1962. The total scheme, with some two million people, is divided into 14 areas that are subdivided into 107 blocks, the basic irrigation units. Several large towns are situated in close proximity to Gezira, e.g., Wad Medani, Hassaheisa and Sennar. Tenant farmers in Gezira live in small villages of about 1000 people each, and there are numerous unregistered villages of *fellata* from Nigeria and immigrants from western Sudan. During the cotton-gathering season many temporary camps are built by seasonal labourers, who may number as many as half a million.

The Gezira-Managil Scheme is one of the largest irrigation projects in Africa. The Sennar Dam, completed in 1925, initially irrigated 105 000 ha, expanding to 336 000 ha by 1950. The Managil Extension brought the cultivated area to 840 000 ha by 1963. These irrigation systems have resulted in a progressive increase in schistosomiasis. The prevalence of *S. haematobium* rose from less than 1% in the period 1924–44 to 21% in adults and 45% in children in 1952. *S. mansoni* prevalences were 5% in 1947, 8.8% in 1952, and between 77% and 86% in children aged 7–9 years in 1973 (Amin, 1977; Omer 1978; Fenwick, 1989).

Since the early 1970s the prevalence of *S. mansoni* has risen while that of *S. haematobium* has decreased. The situation is similar to that in the Nile Delta. By the mid-1970s the prevalence of *S. mansoni* was 73%, whereas that of *S. haematobium* ranged between 1% and 15% and was more focal. An integrated control programme was started in 1979.

The Rahad Scheme, east of the Blue Nile River and covering 126 000 ha, began agricultural activities in 1977–78 and its first phase was completed by 1982. In 1980 the prevalence of *S. mansoni* infection among schoolchildren was 14% and that of *S. haematobium* infection was 1%; in 1988 the corresponding values were 10.3% and 8.5%.

In southern Sudan, Brown et al. (1984) reported that a canal in Bor, taking water from the Nile for use in irrigation, provided a stable habitat for *Bu. truncatus*. The people living near the canal regularly use it as a source of water and it is an important focus of transmission of *S. haematobium*. This finding has serious implications for the projected Jonglei Canal, suggesting the likelihood of new habitats in which *Bu. truncatus* will become established and increase in numbers. This could happen in the main canal if its edges were to become colonized by vegetation or, perhaps more likely, where water is tapped off for irrigation. Increased snail populations, in conjunction with the adoption of a more settled life by the rural Dinka people, could lead to a sharp rise in the prevalence and intensity of infection with urinary schistosomiasis (Southgate, 1984).

Yemen

In Taiz Province, man-made agricultural canals are important foci of transmission, especially associated with the presence of *Biomphalaria pfeifferi*; up to 95% of school-age children are infected and many have hepatosplenomegaly (Hazza et al., 1983).

Region of the Americas

Malaria has been the major parasitic disease associated with water resources development in Latin America (Najera, 1981). Although malaria control has, in general, been successful in Latin America, the development areas within the countries now constitute foci of high incidence and significant morbidity. Malaria spreads between these developments as workers migrate. The risk of schistosomiasis is directly related to the internal migration of labourers from endemic areas in Brazil and Venezuela.

Brazil

Until recently there was little evidence that schistosomiasis was spreading in Brazil as a consequence of water resources development (CNPQ, 1979). An extensive survey of 23 man-made reservoirs and irrigation systems in the states of Ceará, Paraíba, Pernambuco, Piaui, and Rio Grande do Norte in 1979 showed autochthonous cases in São Gonçalo, Paraíba, and Moxotó, Pernambuco (Pereira da Costa & Barbosa, 1985). In 1987 the Ministry of Health reported that the prevalence of the disease in all water resources projects in Piaui, Ceará and Bahía was less than 1% and that the infections that did exist had been acquired elsewhere. In Sergipe, however, infected persons were found in 39 of 54 projects and the prevalence was 24.1%. This was the first indication of the potential for a significant spread of schistosomiasis (PAHO, 1990b).

Paraná-Paraguay Basin

The Itaipu hydroelectric scheme has the potential to produce 12 600 MW through a central dam 1.5 km long and 176 m at maximum height, creating a reservoir of 1460 km^2 (Brasil-Paraguay Itaipu Binacional, 1975). Between 1979 and 1981 more than 100 000 labourers and their families were on site. Before construction, malaria had been reduced to low levels in the area of influence of the dam in Paraguay (there were only six cases in 1976 and 124 in 1975) by effective control and surveillance (PAHO, 1977).

Malaria had been successfully eradicated from southern Brazil but, after the closure of the Itaipu Dam at the end of 1982, the density of *Anopheles darlingi*, the most important vector of malaria in Brazil, began to increase (L. Rey, personal communication, 1989). In 1983, systematic monitoring of the vector was established.

The first 35 autochthonous cases of malaria were registered in 1986; in 1987 and 1988 there were 74 and 157 such cases respectively. In 1989 an epidemic of malaria occurred, 942 autochthonous cases being registered from January to June (nine of which involved *Plasmodium falciparum*). Another 2091 cases involved labourers who had come from the Amazonian Region to Paraguay (PAHO, 1990a). Most of the patients (71%) were found in Foz de Iguaçu. The epidemic peaked in March–April. Although no official data were reported from Paraguay it was estimated that the incidence there was three times greater. Control and surveillance measures were undertaken on one side of the lake, while no intervention took place on the other. Malaria was also reported in Argentina, near the border with Paraguay.

Biomphalaria straminea, one of the intermediate snail hosts of *Schistosoma mansoni*, was found in Itaipu before the dam was built, but autochthonous transmission has not yet been detected despite high snail population densities. *Bi. glabrata* exists elsewhere in the basin some 500 km from the lake.

São Francisco Basin

Schistosomiasis is the principal parasitic disease risk. The prevalence in the area of the man-made lakes in Barreiras and São Desiderio, Bahía, is 18.5%, and in the area of Betume Dam, Sergipe, it is over 25%. In the development areas of the States of Bahía, Sergipe and Alagoas, visceral leishmaniasis is endemic and presents an important health risk for the associated settlements.

Amazon Basin

In this region the construction is under way of the Balbina Dam, which will create a large man-made lake. Malaria is highly endemic and control can be seen only as a long-term goal. Multiplication of the breeding places of *Anopheles darlingi* is a threat in all Amazonian lakes. The arrival of workers from areas of Brazil where the disease is not endemic creates dramatic epidemic foci. More than half a million cases a year occur in gold-mining areas and new agricultural zones.

Schistosomiasis, previously limited to a few endemic foci in the Salgado region and to the two extinguished foci of Fordlandia and Belterra on the Tapajos River, is now an important problem in the city of Belém where *Biomphalaria glabrata* is rapidly multiplying under houses built on wooden piles over water and occupied by poor immigrant families. *Bi. amazonica* is also widespread in the Amazon region, and is capable of transmitting *S. mansoni*.

Other arthropod-borne infections of relevance in this large equatorial region are leishmaniasis, yellow fever, viral encephalitis and certain other viral diseases, as well as onchocerciasis (in the north-central part of the region) and lymphatic filariasis (in the east); the incidence of these diseases is influenced by the density of their insect vectors.

Araguaia-Tocantins Basin

Because there was no deforestation in the 2430-km^2 area of the reservoir of the Tucurui Dam on the Tocantins river, eutrophication created ideal conditions for the extensive growth of floating vegetation (*Salvinia auriculata*). This supported the proliferation of *Mansonia titillans*, an aggressive culicine mosquito with a painful bite for both man and cattle. The people living near the shores abandoned their land and moved elsewhere.

Suriname

Between 1903 and 1912 the construction of the railway from Paramaribo to the Saracreek Dam was interrupted several times by malaria epidemics among the labourers. In 1905 up to 50% of the labourers from Curaçao had malaria and all survivors were repatriated. In 1906, 200 labourers from Barbados replaced them, but all returned home after one year (Oostberg, 1977).

In the Brokopondo Dam projects the resettlement of local residents from the flooded areas and the introduction of irrigation have increased the risks of vector-borne diseases. Although malaria is endemic, the provision of local health services and transportation of patients to other health facilities has kept it under control (Oostberg, 1977).

South-East Asia and Western Pacific Regions

In Asia, there is relatively little evidence of adverse health effects of water resources. Sornmani & Harinasuta (1988) have pointed out that the health care infrastructure, the level of local commitment to development, and certain biological characteristics of the arthropod and snail vectors, militate against excessive short-term health effects.

Since 1980 *Schistosoma malayensis* has been confirmed as a human parasite with *Robertsiella kaporensis* as its intermediate host; this hydrobiid snail predominantly inhabits the root masses of *Saraca thaipingensis* in rapidly flowing waters. The parasite has a wild reservoir in the rat *Rattus muelleri* (Greer et al., 1980). This is a zoonotic infection and is unlikely to become a significant public health problem (Greer et al., 1989).

The spread of schistosomiasis in relation to water resources development has not been documented in Asia. However, projects such as the Gumbasa Irrigation Project in Indonesia, the Phitsanulok Irrigation Project in Thailand and the Pahang River Basin Project in Malaysia are located in areas where schistosomiasis has been reported. In addition, such projects merit surveillance for the fish-borne trematode infections, clonorchiasis and opisthorchiasis. The development of the basin of the Mun River, a tributary of the Mekong River in north-east Thailand, could give rise to a focus of schistosomiasis (Sornmani & Harinasuta, 1988).

Where filariasis is endemic, as in the Baritos River Basin Development Project in Indonesia, the Bicol River Basin Development Project in the Philippines, and the Pahang River Basin Project in Malaysia, there is clearly a high risk of increased prevalence and severity of the disease.

India

Malaria has become highly endemic in the Raichur district of Karnataka State following the construction of the Tungabhadra Dam and the associated canal network (Centre for Science and Ecology, 1982).

In villages along the irrigation canals of the Meerut District of Uttar Pradesh, rates of malaria are six times greater in June and nine times greater in October than those in villages of Guragon District in Haryana State which are 40 km from canals (Centre for Science and Ecology, 1985).

In the 1940s the Malaria Institute of India emphasized that the perennial irrigation projects in Punjab, Uttar Pradesh and Sind would extend mosquito habitats, thus causing the prevalence of malaria to increase (Centre for Science and Ecology, 1982).

In Koraput District, Orissa State, the highest prevalence of malaria was observed in a workers' camp attached to an irrigation project site. The prevalence among the migrant labourers was nearly 40%, compared with 20% among the local people, *P. falciparum* being predominant (Rajagopalan, 1990).

Philippines

Schistosomiasis remains the major public health challenge in irrigation systems in the Philippines (Blas, 1989). It has been estimated that 25% of the transmission of *S. japonicum* to people is due to contamination of the environment by infected wild rodents (Blas, 1976).

Sri Lanka

The Mahaweli River flows for 315 km from central Sri Lanka to the east coast. Five major dams were constructed between 1970 and 1976, and more are under construction (Alexis, 1986). In 1986–87 malaria outbreaks due to *P. falciparum* occurred for the first time upstream from the Victoria Dam. Resistance to chloroquine complicated control measures: 53% of patients had four or more attacks within the survey period. The increased incidence of malaria has been variously explained by (1) the movement of migrants with malaria into project areas, (2) the low river discharge leading to the formation of pools, thus promoting mosquito breeding, and (3) a change of hosts by *A. culicifacies* from animals to man as agricultural mechanization reduces the need for buffalos on farms (Samarasinghe, 1986; Wijesundera, 1988).

Thailand and Lao People's Democratic Republic

In Thailand the prevalence of opisthorchiasis (liver fluke disease transmitted to humans through the consumption of raw freshwater fish) was higher among residents of the Nam Pong Resources Development Project than among people in surrounding nonirrigated areas. Irrigation creates snail habitats and leads to increases in fish populations, producing a high rate of transmission where there is contamination with human faeces. Furthermore, fish from this area are sold over the whole region, thus increasing the spread of infection among populations at some distance from the project.

Sornmani & Harinasuta (1988) noted reports of high morbidity and mortality due to malaria among skilled workers during construction of the Nam Ngum Dam in Lao People's Democratic Republic and the Quae Yai Multipurpose Project in Thailand.

In Thailand the artificial lake in the Srinagarind Water Resources Development Project destroyed breeding sites of *Anopheles dirus* but populations of *Culex tritaeniorhyncus*, the vector of Japanese encephalitis, increased.

Rice fields are major habitats for rats, whose numbers may become astronomical and produce adverse consequences for human health. In the Phitsanulok Irrigation Project in Central Thailand nearly 50% of field rats were found to be infected with *Schistosoma incognitum*. This parasite does not reach maturity in man despite penetration of the skin but it became a major cause of dermatitis and of lost working time among Thai farmers.

European Region

The former USSR

Dramatic increases in diphyllobothriasis, a fish tapeworm that produces severe anaemia, have been associated with large reservoirs in the Volga-Kama Basin, the Enisei Basin, and the Bratsk and Krasnoyarsk Reservoirs in Siberia. In the Volgograd region, before the construction of a large reservoir, the prevalence of diphyllobothriasis was low; after the filling of the reservoir, however, the prevalence reached 25% in some villages. At the Kuibyshevskoye and Permskoye Reservoirs, prevalence rose to 48%. No infection was present for the first few years after dam construction in the Enisei Basin, but the prevalence is now increasing yearly. Around Bratskoye Reservoir, 48% of the population are infected, while at Krasnoyarskoye the highest prevalence is 12% (Iarotski & Pluscheva, 1989).

In the Irghiz–Turghai region, opisthorchiasis is highly endemic. However, the construction of the Irtysh–Karaganda–Djezkazghan canal, which incorporates several reservoirs, has reduced the prevalence of the disease. This is a result of: (1) changes in fish populations, reducing the intermediate fish hosts of the parasite, (2) salination, (3) drainage of part of the watershed, (4) reduction of rodent reservoir hosts, and (5) decreased contamination of water by sewage effluents (Iarotski & Pluscheva, 1989).

The E. I. Martsinovsky Institute, Moscow, in collaboration with the Ministry of Health, maintains ecological and health surveillance of 20 large reservoirs in the Dnieper, Volga, Kama, Don, Daugava, Enisei, Ob, Seya, and Amu-Darya River Basins (Iarotski & Pluscheva, 1989). Among the people residing around these reservoirs, diphyllobothriasis and opisthorchiasis are important public health problems.

Turkey

The large irrigation schemes of Seyhan I (65 000 ha) and Seyhan II (42 300 ha), begun in 1963 and associated with the Seyhan, Berdan and Ceyhan Rivers in southern Anatolia, could eventually extend to 181 000 ha on the Çukurova Plains. The uncontrolled influx of migrant workers, estimated to number 200 000 in 1962 and about 700 000 in 1976, brought *P. vivax* from surrounding malarious areas. This was the single most important epidemiological factor in the ensuing malaria epidemic (Giglioli, 1979).

Throughout the irrigation system there was poor water management and silting problems for which machinery was not available. The older Seyhan scheme remained unrehabilitated. Tertiary drainage canals were cleaned only once every 5–6 years rather than every 3 years, and main drainage canals were cleaned at intervals of 7–8 years instead of every 4–5 years. Herbicides were used on a limited scale or not at all (State Water Works, unpublished report, 1981). Thus mosquito habitats were undisturbed and control of the indigenous *Anopheles* species had ceased by 1965.

These environmental and epidemiological factors, coupled with the failure of the public health surveillance system, led to disaster. In 1976 and 1977 there were 37 200 and 115 512 reported cases of *P. vivax* infection, respectively (Clarke, 1982), of which 101 649 were in the Çukurova and Amikova regions (Giglioli, 1979), and a national emergency was declared.

Need for vigilance in projects currently under development

The Introduction highlighted an encouraging trend to include health considerations in project planning. This section describes some current or proposed water resource development projects. In most, the impact of parasitic diseases has yet to be studied. In some projects, assessment has been undertaken before impoundment, surveillance of vectors and parasitic diseases has been instituted, and adequate health care delivery has been provided for personnel and, occasionally, for the surrounding populations. The experience gained should provide an indication of the seriousness with which economic development planners take their responsibilities towards human health. Each situation provides a challenge for national health services to participate actively in the development process.

Angola: Capanda Dam

The Capanda Dam on the Kwanza River was due to be completed in 1992, creating an artificial lake with a volume of 3.7 km^3 and providing irrigation for 120 000 ha (GAMEK, 1988). During the construction phase, all workers are being screened for urinary schistosomiasis and all infected persons are being treated (Barbosa, 1990). Malaria has been reduced by chemoprophylaxis and mosquito control, and African sleeping sickness, which is endemic in the region, is effectively controlled by *Glossina* fly traps. The close collaboration between the construction enterprise and the endemic disease control services of the Ministry of Health is exemplary. However, there is apparently no long-term fiscal and organizational provision for post-construction health maintenance.

Brazil: São Francisco Valley

The São Francisco Valley Development Company (CODEVASF) is in charge of the planning and implementation of irrigation projects. Through its initiative and financing, 216 900 ha were cultivated in 1988, of which 127 500 ha were irrigated. To date, 32 medium-size or small dams have been constructed for irrigation, and another 13 have been built to provide domestic water supplies. CODEVASF has plans to irrigate another 123 000 ha in the next few years.

All of these projects include studies of potential health problems and the design of a health services infrastructure capable of responding to the situation.

For health maintenance, CODEVASF constructed a hospital with 33 beds, and 61 health centres in five states. The operation of health services was transferred to the Foundation for Special Public Health Services (FSESP), but no project funds were made available for health maintenance. As of 1984, only 45 health centres were open and the hospital was still empty. This is a case of infrastructural development being left without financial support. A special agreement has now been made to transfer control, responsibility and funds to SUCAM (Public Health Campaign, Ministry of Health). These organizational changes release the initiating development agency from any financial or other responsibility for health. In the São Francisco Valley, the important endemic diseases that are likely to be influenced by the new ecological conditions are schistosomiasis, malaria, yellow fever and Chagas disease (CODEVASF, 1989).

China: Three Gorges Project

A review of the potential impact of schistosomiasis and malaria around an 800 km^2 lake to be created by a proposed dam at the Three Gorges site has been completed by the Institute of Parasitic Diseases of the Sichuan Provincial Academy of Medical Sciences (Gu et al., 1988). Schistosomiasis due to *S. japonicum* is not endemic in the area, and the immersion of habitats of the uninfected snail *Oncomelania* should eliminate any danger from this quarter. The distance to the nearest area of endemicity upstream in Sichuan or Yunnan Provinces is 500 km, but the nearest downstream focus in Hubei Province, where the disease is highly endemic, is only 80 km away at the beginning of the lake region of the Chang (Yangtze) River Basin.

The late Professor Su De-Long of Shanghai First Medical University was unable to find any schistosomiasis in the Xin an Jiang Reservoir in Zhejiang Province or in the Dongzhang Reservoir in Fujian. Longitudinal surveys of six reservoirs in different areas of endemicity in Jiangsu Province, conducted by Professor Zhao Weixian of Nanjing Medical College, indicated that *Oncomelania* snails tended to disappear two years after water impoundment.

It was concluded that schistosomiasis was not prevalent in the Three Gorges area to be inundated and that nearby upstream areas of endemicity did not constitute a significant risk to the reservoir site, but that schistosomiasis was endemic downstream, that suitable conditions existed for *Oncomelania* habitats, and that careful field studies and surveillance of transmission were necessary.

Another report highlighted the potential impact of the Three Gorges Project on malaria (Chen et al., 1989). It was noted that malaria had once been highly endemic in the area, and that three major epidemics had occurred between 1881 and 1919.

Accurate records on malaria are available only for the recent past. In 1988 the incidence of the disease in the 26 counties of the proposed site was 2.2 per 10 000; 34.7% of the townships were malaria-free, and 6.5% had incidence rates exceeding 10 per 10 000. *Anopheles sinensis* was the dominant vector (95.3%) and anopheline larvae were observed only in the Changshaba and Hulukou Reservoirs. No malaria infection was reported in local residents. Two surveys of the Gongzui and Shizitan Reservoirs did not find *Anopheles*.

It was concluded that: (1) there was a potential risk of malaria outbreaks during construction of the dam; (2) malaria might be spread by migrants leaving the impoundment area; (3) *Anopheles* was more likely to breed in the tributaries of the river than in the lake itself; and (4) the potential impact of malaria on local residents after the completion of the dam should not be ignored because of its bearing on future economic development.

The World Food Programme has been approached to consider providing food aid support to the following projects, which indicate the extensive range of water resources development in China.

- 1980—Construction of reservoirs and reclamation of waste land at Binchuan Farm, Yunnan Province.
- 1981—Development of fishery resources in Hongze County, Jiangsu Province.
- 1983—Agricultural development through improved drainage and irrigation in Anhui Province.
- 1983—Development of aquaculture in low-lying saline alkaline lands, Hangzhou Bay, Zhejiang Province.
- 1984—Development of coastal aquaculture in Bohai Bay, Shandong and Hebei Provinces.
- 1985—Aquaculture in ten cities.
- 1987—Agricultural development through irrigation, Wulan County, Qinghai Province.
- 1988—Comprehensive development of mountainous areas in three counties of Guangxi Zhuang Autonomous Region.
- 1988—Comprehensive development of mountainous areas in Shexian County, Hubei Province.
- 1988—Integrated agricultural developments in the Wuling Mountains, Hunan and Hubei Provinces.
- 1988—Agricultural development through irrigation, Jintaichuan Command area, Gansu Province.
- 1989—Integrated agricultural development, Yunnan Province.

WHO collaborated with the World Food Programme in assessing the likely health impact of parasitic diseases before support was given for each project. Intestinal parasitic infections are endemic in all the project areas. In coastal areas and southern parts of the country, trematode infections, such as clonorchiasis, may be associated with aquaculture development. Schistosomiasis is generally well controlled in China except in the central part of the Chang (Yangtze) River Basin, bordered by Hunan and Hubei provinces (WHO, 1988). In most of the areas of the projects supported by the World Food Programme, schistosomiasis is either not endemic or is under surveillance.

Ethiopia

According to the central planning office of the Supreme Council in 1984 (Tedla et al., 1989), 14 river basins including the Blue Nile, Baro-Akobo, Awash, Mereb-Gash, Barka, Omo and Wabi-Shebelle, provide an irrigated land potential of 1.82 million ha in more than 50 project areas. Since 1979 no fewer than 44 irrigation schemes have been planned or completed, covering a total of over 500 000 ha. Most are in the north of the country where few schemes currently exist. Many of the irrigated farms will be settled, at least partially, by victims of the drought from Welo, Gondar, Tigray and Hararge. These are areas of high endemicity for schistosomiasis and the settlers could spread the disease. Existing schemes are concentrated in the Awash Valley and in the Hararge and Welo Regions (Tedla et al., 1989).

India: Narmada Valley

During the last three decades the pace of dam construction in India has accelerated and by October 1989 about 1600 dams of varying sizes had been built. The Narmada Valley Project is the biggest of the river valley projects so far proposed.

The Narmada is the largest west-flowing river in India. It rises in the highlands of eastern Madhya Pradesh and flows in a narrow valley for 1300 km, draining an area of 98 800 km^2 before discharging into the Gulf of Cambay. Its average annual flow is 45 000 million m^3, more than the combined flows of the Ravi, Beas, and Sutlej, which feed the Indus Basin. More than 90% of the run-off occurs between June and September, the monsoon season, so that its effective utilization requires the construction of large reservoirs. Comprehensive plans for the development of the Narmada River include thirty major projects. The Sardar Sarovar hydroelectric scheme is designed to generate 1450 MW of electricity and irrigate 1 870 000 ha, including drought-prone and poor areas of Gujarat, by the early 1990s. The main irrigation canal will have one of the world's largest capacities for water supply, at 1130 m^3/sec, and will transport water 439 km as far as the Rajasthan border. The 370-km^2 reservoir will occupy 20 822 ha in Madhya Pradesh and Maharashtra, and most of the

70 000 people who will be displaced live in that area (Indian Insti Management, 1989).

The Narmada Sagar Irrigation and Power Complex in Madhya ι desh consists potentially of three large dams with hydropower faciliti Narmada Sagar (1000 MW), Omkareshwar (400 MW) and Maheshwar (200 MW) on the lower Narmada River. These dams should provide irrigation for some 300 000 ha, together with domestic and industrial water.

The Narmada Sagar Project, under appraisal since 1985, will create the largest man-made lake in India and will cause the largest population resettlement to date of any scheme that has been assisted by the World Bank. This project consists mainly of a reservoir of 91 350 ha (of which about 35 000 ha are currently forest, 31 000 ha are private farmland, and the remainder is private or public grazing and waste land). It will entail the resettlement of about 85 000 people from 253 villages and a town in Madhya Pradesh. Approximately 40 000 ha of forest will be planted to compensate for the area to be inundated. The afforestation and resettle-ment components will be companion projects. Work on the 142-km^2 Omkareshwar Reservoir and the 49-km^2 Maheshwar Reservoir is not yet firmly scheduled, but should start about two years after work begins on the Narmada Sagar Project. These two sites would irrigate 175 000 ha. An area of 156 000 ha would be irrigated by the Narmada Sagar (World Bank Joint Mission, 1985).

A recent reappraisal of the distribution of schistosomiasis suggests there is a real threat that it will spread (Southgate & Agrawal, 1990). Clear provisions have not yet been made to secure the maintenance of health in the Narmada Valley Project. The World Bank delayed approval for the project on environmental grounds; whether this explicitly ad-dressed risks to human health is not clear (Goodland, 1989). On the other hand, malaria has been effectively controlled in India and should not represent a major risk (Goodland, 1985).

Kenya: Seven Forks Scheme

The first dam in the Seven Forks Scheme, Kindaruma, was begun in 1963 and completed in 1968. It was followed by the Kamburu in 1975 and the Gitaru, situated between them, in 1979 (Oomen, 1981). The Masinga dam was begun in 1978 and completed in 1980. The Bura irrigation scheme, covering 6700 ha in its first stage of development, is only 45 km north of the Hola irrigation scheme, which is highly endemic for schistosomiasis (Oomen, 1981). As this area continues to develop, all parasitic diseases are likely to be major health problems.

Malaysia: Nenggiri Dam

The proposed Nenggiri Hydroelectric Power Project is located on the Nenggiri River at Kg Setar, 25 km north of Gua Musang town and near the centre of the South Kelantan Development Authority Project. The dam will inundate an area of 10 900 ha, requiring resettlement of slightly over 2000 persons including those in 25 aboriginal settlements. Malaria has been the major problem in the area. The mosquito vectors of filariasis and dengue are present. Schistosomiasis has been reported among the aboriginal Orang Asli people in the area. The low level of literacy, the loss of land, and resettlement without adequate water supplies and sanitation could lead to extensive health problems (Taib, 1989).

Mauritania: Gorgol Rice Irrigation System

Two proposed dams on the Gorgol River will create the lower El-Bir and the upper Foum Gleita Reservoirs. Malaria and urinary schistosomiasis were endemic over the entire area from Kaedi at the junction of the Gorgol and Senegal Rivers to the upper reaches of the proposed Foum Gleita Reservoir. The situation was assessed and comprehensive recommendations were made on the design and management of the system with a view to mitigating the consequences of parasitic diseases (Oomen et al., 1988).

Myanmar: Sedawgyi Multipurpose and Irrigation Project

The Sedawgyi Dam site is located on the Chaung-magyi River in Madaya township, 46 miles north-east of Mandalay City. It is expected to provide irrigation for 125 000 ha and 25 MW from a reservoir approximately 60 km^2 in area. Malaria was the main health problem during the deforestation and construction phase in 1984, when there were 144 087 cases of malaria and 26 deaths from the disease; since then the numbers have halved (Aung Tun Thet, 1989).

Niger: Kandadji Dam

Kandadji Dam will be built on the Niger River near the border with Mali, 11 km from Ayorou and 566 km from Niamey. It will provide irrigation for 100 000 ha and produce about 360 000 MWh of electricity per year (Niger, 1980). The prevalence of urinary schistosomiasis in the area is as high as 94% in some villages (Doumenge et al., 1987).

Rwanda: Kagara River Basin Development Project

The Rusumo, Murongo and Kakono Dams form the major part of the proposed Kagara River Basin Development Project. Planning has been under way for many years but implementation has been delayed. Malaria is highly endemic in this region. The prevalence of schistosomiasis is low; however, the snail intermediate host is found throughout the Kagara River Basin fish ponds (Malek 1983) and in the irrigation schemes between the Muvumbu and Kakituma rivers (Ohse, 1980). Migration of infected people from the Rusizi Plains in Burundi and the West Lake Region of the United Republic of Tanzania indicates a high risk of transmission (Gigase & Hanotier, 1982).

Senegal: Senegal Valley

Malaria is prevalent in this area. Large swamps and lakes near the river banks provide breeding places for mosquitos. Rice irrigation projects, if not correctly managed, will allow permanent, year-round mosquito breeding. Water infiltration and poor drainage of impoundments will produce mosquito infestations.

Not only will the transmission of malaria and schistosomiasis be favoured, but zoonotic leishmaniasis, of which there was recently an epidemic, will be sustained by important rodent and phlebotomine populations in a more permanent ecological context.

Two major water development projects, the Manantali and Diama Dams, were recently denied funding by the World Bank, partly on environmental grounds (Goodland, 1989). This action appears to have been justified since schistosomiasis and malaria are now major problems (Talla et al., 1990).

Somalia: Juba Valley

Health impact studies have been made for the proposed hydroelectric scheme in the Juba River Valley. The lake will permit a number of irrigation projects, such as the Juba Sugar Project (6500 ha with sprinkler irrigation over 92% of the area), the Fanoole Rice Project (now 630 ha, with a potential of 48 000 ha), and the Mogambo Irrigation Project (500 ha). *S. haematobium* is prevalent throughout the Juba Valley, especially below Baadhere.

The initial step in evaluating health risks was to estimate the extent of aquatic habitats to be expected within and around the proposed lake. This

provides a basis for predicting insect and snail populations and the potential for disease transmission under varying conditions of the reservoir and
human settlement. It has been estimated that snail densities will he highest
during the autumn, and that this will cause increased schistosomiasis
transmission during the autumn and winter (Jobin, 1989).

The expected transmission pattern of malaria was also considered. The
reservoir is expected to be full during the autumn, when it is likely that
Anopheles funestus will inhabit the shore and cause a new period of malaria
transmission. This will reduce the gap between the two main malaria
seasons caused by *A. gambiae*. and may result in year-round transmission.

Environmental management of the shoreline could reduce malaria
transmission and contribute to the control of other diseases (Jobin, 1989).

South Africa

In a recent review of 95 South African dams it was concluded that all
those within areas of endemicity posed a risk of transmission of urinary
and/or intestinal schistosomiasis (Pretorius et al., 1989).

Sudan: Jonglei Canal

In southern Sudan, Brown et al. (1984) reported the presence of
Bu. truncatus and the transmission of *S. haematobium* in a canal at Bor. This
finding has serious implications in that the Jonglei Canal can be expected
to provide new habitats allowing *Bu. truncatus* to become established and
increase in numbers, possibly in the main canal where the edges are
colonized by vegetation and especially where water is tapped off for
irrigation. Increased snail populations, and the adoption of a more settled
life by the rural Dinka people, could lead to a sharp rise in the prevalence
and intensity of infection of urinary schistosomiasis.

Turkey: south-east Anatolian Project

The proposed development project in south-east Anatolia would create 18
artificial lakes and two conveyance tunnels on the upper Euphrates and
Tigris Rivers and would permit the irrigation of 1 800 000 ha. On the
upper Euphrates the Keban Dam is completed, one is under construction
at Karakaya, and a third at Karababa will provide irrigation for the Urfa
Plain. Proximity to areas where schistosomiasis is endemic in both Turkey
and the Syrian Arab Republic and the high prevalence of malaria, do not
augur well for the health impact of this project. In 1970 there were about

70 irrigation reservoirs in Turkey and by the year 2000 there will be over 100.

United Republic of Tanzania: Rufiji Basin Development Project

The Rufiji River is formed by the confluence of the Luwegu and Kilombero Rivers. The Rufiji River Basin covers about 20% of the country's surface area and is inhabited by 10% of its population. The Rufiji Basin Development Authority was established in 1975 and proposed a multipurpose scheme, the Steigler's Gorge Power and Flood Control Project. The dam at Steigler's Gorge will provide flood control and a reservoir covering a third of the Rufiji district, allowing the irrigation of at least 64 900 ha. Urinary schistosomiasis was present in villages that were to be inundated but its prevalance was below 10%. Only *Bulinus nasutus* and *Bulinus globosus* were found in the 78 bodies of water which were investigated. The proposed project would stabilize and extend the habitats of the intermediate snail hosts and protect them from the effects of seasonal drought. Intensified year-round transmission of schistosomiasis would probably ensue (Mwanza, 1982).

Zaire: Mobayi-Mbongo Dam

A dam across the Ubangi River was completed at Mobayi-Mbongo in Equator Province in mid-1989. In 1967 prevalences of under 1% of both urinary and intestinal schistosomiasis were observed, but in the last 20 years the disease has increased, probably as a result of the arrival of infected workers from Bas-Zaïre. By early 1989, surveys in villages along the river revealed that the prevalence of urinary and intestinal schistosomiasis in children was greater below than above the dam site. Downstream the prevalence of *S. haematobium* and *S. mansoni* infection was 32% and 15% respectively (Delbaère, 1989). As economic development proceeds following construction of a hydroelectric power plant, it is probable that disease levels will rise further in people of all ages, yet the local health services have not been expanded.

4.

Health effects of small village dams

Disease intensification

Public attention is focused on the large water development projects of the tropical world because of their intrinsic scientific and engineering interest and their symbolic value for human achievement. However, it is likely that small impoundments, in their totality, have an equally great or even greater significance for human health (Hunter et al., 1980, 1982). In Nigeria and Zimbabwe, for instance, the shore length of small impoundments has been estimated to be 8–10 times that of the large reservoirs (Jewsbury & Imevbore, 1988).

Small impoundments tend to serve more purposes than large dams. A small multipurpose project may be used for fishing, water supplies, watering of cattle and livestock, irrigation, and flood control. Usually there is a high degree of contact with water by people and animals, so that disease transmission rates, especially for zoonoses, are considerable. Small multipurpose village dams, together with clusters of fish ponds, have a great potential for intensifying and spreading disease. Small impoundments, although undoubtedly of benefit to agriculture, are also hazardous to health, while health care provision is usually inadequate.

The creation of a small dam may convert the prevailing, scattered, relatively low-level endemicity into localized hyperendemicity. Cercarial density and frequency of water contact per unit of shoreline and per unit volume of water are usually greater in small impoundments than in large lakes. Small impoundments can thus rapidly become intense foci of schistosomiasis transmission. The breeding of blackflies in the spillways of small dams during the rainy season means that onchocerciasis is a severe threat to surrounding populations. The incidence and prevalence of malaria, lymphatic filariasis, and dracunculiasis are also increased around small dams. Severe forms of these diseases, especially lymphatic filariasis (elephantiasis), may occur frequently because of the intensity of transmission (Hunter, 1992).

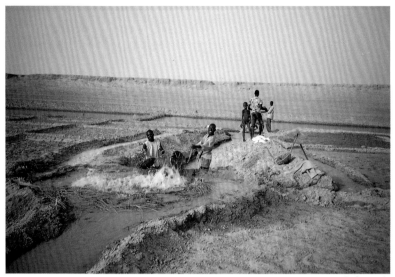

Artisanal irrigation systems in the Niger Delta area of Mali are widespread and associated with high prevalences of malaria and schistosomiasis.

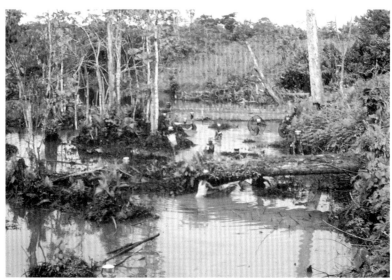

Tin strip-mining creates extensive breeding sites for mosquitos and freshwater snails. In these conditions in Maniema, Zaire, the transmission of intestinal schistosomiasis due to *S. mansoni* and of malaria is intense.

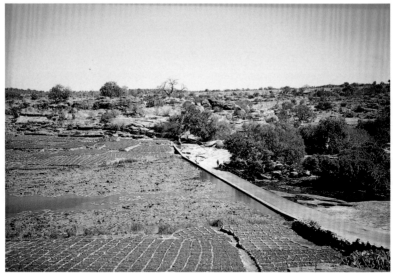

B. Gryseels

In arid regions of Africa, as in the Dogon plateau of Mali, small reservoirs and their irrigation systems are intense foci of transmission of schistosomiasis and malaria.

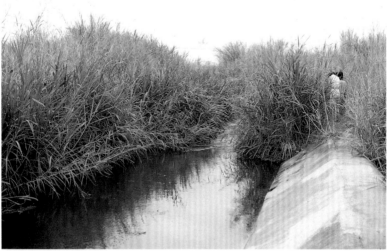

C. Lengler

Concrete lining of irrigation canals does not eliminate the potential for breeding of either mosquitos or freshwater snails. Systematic maintenance is required.

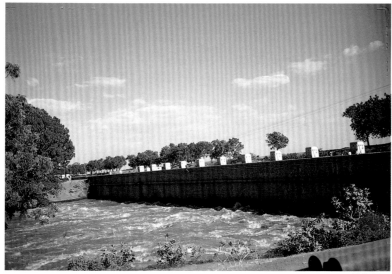

K. E. Mott

The Sennar dam, completed in 1925, initiated the Gezira-Mangil irrigation system, the largest single irrigation system in the world. Increased prevalences of malaria and schistosomasis ensued, and remain major public health problems.

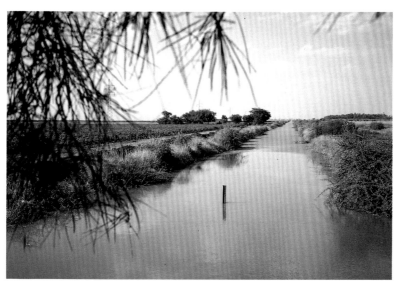

K. E. Mott

Maintenance of unlined irrigation canals would help to increase agricultural productivity and to reduce the breeding of mosquitos and freshwater snails.

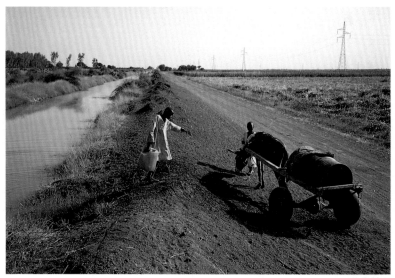

Safe domestic water supplies, as part of the basic infrastructure of any water resources development scheme, could help avoid scenes like this.

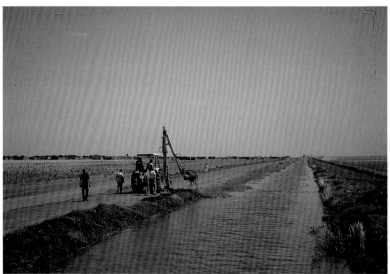

In large irrigation schemes, mechanical clearance of vegetation from the canals is necessary for optimum production, and also reduces snail habitats.

To date, however, no systematic investigation has been made into the problems of disease transmission in small, man-made bodies of water. There is a scarcity of studies on disease elevation around small village dams in tropical regions. This poses a regrettable information gap for health care authorities. Investigations are few, and most of those that have been conducted have compared disease prevalence in the area of a dam with that at a distance. There have been no strictly controlled epidemiological studies of pre- and post-impoundment prevalence and intensity of transmission. However, all the available information unequivocally associates dams with serious increases in disease. Some illustrations are given below.

Cameroon

In addition to some medium-sized dams built in Cameroon about 20 years ago, large numbers of small dams have been built in the last 10 years, as well as over 100 small artificial lakes for fish culture. Some of the earthworks provide for irrigated rice growing. These developments have led to considerable increases in the prevalence of schistosomiasis, onchocerciasis, dracunculiasis and malaria (Ripert & Raccurt, 1987; E. A. Malek, personal communication, 1989).

Ghana

The prevalence of onchocerciasis (river blindness) has been observed to increase with the crowding of populations around progressively diminishing water bodies during drought (Hunter, 1966, 1967a,b). USAID constructed 104 small dams in north-east Ghana between 1958 and 1960, to provide community water supplies, support livestock, and irrigate vegetable gardens in the dry season. Although onchocerciasis has indeed decreased—probably as a result of effective vector control— an analysis in 38 survey areas indicated that the median prevalence of schistosomiasis caused by S. haematobium tripled from 17% to 50.5% as a result of the constructions. The disease reached levels of 70% in some areas. Today, many of these dams are derelict as a result of excessive silting, spillway damage and the breaching of impoundment walls.

When these small dams were built, 30 years ago, no measures for disease prevention were introduced. Today there is a proposal to construct about 120 new dams and rehabilitate 100 old ones in the same area. Regrettably, no budgetary provisions have been made for health protection, without which further disease outbreaks can be expected (Hunter, 1981).

Kenya

In Kenya, small irrigation schemes are independently managed and do not come under the jurisdiction of the National Irrigation Board. They take water from rivers and streams, some of which are highly infected with *S. mansoni*. A programme of registration and control is needed for such schemes (P. Jordan, personal communication, 1989).

In Nyanza Province some 10 000 ponds were dug with the aim of increasing fish production. They resulted in considerable breeding of malaria vectors. No assessment of the impact on public health has been made but Masaba et al. (1983) reported that focal prevalence of *S. haematobium* exceeded 30% and that haematuria occurred frequently in schoolchildren in two villages located near some of the ponds.

Mali

Urinary schistosomiasis is endemic throughout the Cercle de Bandiagara, where about 20 small dams had been completed by 1977. No surveys were made before this work started, but a comparison of data for a population in 1976 and 1977 showed an increase in the prevalence of schistosomiasis from 79.4% to 93.4% (Scott & Chu, 1977). In addition, local transmission of *S. mansoni* was demonstrated for the first time in the 1977 survey. It can be concluded that the barrage system has probably led to an increase in transmission.

Surveys carried out by the *Organisation de Coordination et de Coopération pour la Lutte contre les Grandes Endémies* (OCCGE) have demonstrated high levels of schistosomiasis associated with the cultivation of rice along the flood plain of the Niger.

More recently, surveys of 34 434 people in 225 villages in different ecological settings with both large- and small-scale irrigation showed, as expected, that areas of rice and sugar irrigation had high prevalences, especially of serious intestinal disease; similar prevalences were reported in localities with small dams (Brinkmann et al., 1988). The prevalence of urinary schistosomiasis was five times greater in villages with small dams (67%) than among savanna villages (13%). Intestinal schistosomiasis showed a similar pattern (see Table 11, page 38).

Rwanda

In 1983 an inspection of fish ponds that had been constructed in the prefectures of Butare, Gikongoro, Gitarama, Gisenyi and Kigali revealed the presence of the snail hosts of *S. mansoni* (*Biomphalaria pfeifferi* and *Bi.*

sudanica) and those of *S. haematobium* (*Bulinus globosus*). Although no infection with *S. mansoni* or *S. haematobium* was found in these snails, their presence suggested the possibility of schistosomiasis transmission (Malek, 1983).

Zambia

Many small dams in Zambia are snail-free. However, snails (particularly *Biomphalaria* spp.) are often abundant in seepages below the walls of dams in areas where people have small vegetable gardens. In these circumstances there is a high risk of transmission (R. F. Sturrock, personal communication, 1989).

Rapid construction rate of small dams

Countless small dams have been constructed both privately and by local authorities in recent decades, and it is likely that the rate of construction is increasing rapidly. The registration of dams less than 15 m in height is not within the scope of the International Commission on Large Dams. Exceptionally some dams 10–15 m high may be registered. National registration is usually not required, so numbers and locations are often unknown by administrative and planning authorities. Small dams may be built by local authorities with government support, or by nongovernmental organizations, missionary societies, chiefs and local community groups.

One reason for the growing numbers of small dams and impoundments has been the increased availability of earth-moving equipment for both official and private purposes. This has allowed village communities and farmers' cooperatives to proceed with construction on their own initiative. Road contractors with heavy equipment may be hired privately to do such work. Especially when small dams are not government-financed, there are problems of maintenance, seepage, and discipline in water use, all of which favour the extension of vector habitats. The dams serve to exacerbate disease transmission, regardless of whether the agronomic outcomes are favourable or poor.

Registration of small dams

Small dams that, individually, may be overlooked by health planners become big in aggregate. Bilateral and multilateral assistance programmes generate much of the expansion under the aegis of economic development. For example, USAID has constructed some 50 village dams in Cameroon and over 100 in Ghana, in relatively dense regional clusters. Canada and Germany are considering further support for dam construction in Ghana. Given the acute need for water for livestock, agriculture and community use in dry tropical areas, it is certain that the construction of impoundments will continue.

This constitutes an ominous but overlooked threat to health, and presents a potential focus for intersectoral collaboration. The compilation and maintenance of national registers of water impoundments could be used in integrated health planning of preventive measures and disease control in high-risk areas. Registration or simplified listing would draw attention to the importance of small lakes and impoundments and indicate the scale of the challenge to health. Because of the cost and, more importantly, the infrastructural significance for other sectors of government, registration would have to be broadly intersectoral.

Although there is a lack of information at the central levels of government on the distribution of small dams, health workers and agricultural extension personnel at the local level have a thorough knowledge of the subject. The task of recording the existence of small impoundments could be done through a district-level reporting system, originating at the village level with health aides or agricultural extension agents. The information could then be incorporated into a national list on a cumulative basis. The use of aerial photography and remote sensing, integrated into a geographical information system, is a further possibility.

5.

Disease control in water development schemes

The control of parasitic diseases is a daunting challenge. One or more of the commonest of these diseases—filariasis, malaria, onchocerciasis and schistosomiasis—are endemic in each of the 41 least-developed countries, as designated by the United Nations. All four diseases are endemic in 16 of the 24 least-developed countries in Africa. Constraints on disease control include shortage of trained national staff and lack of financial resources (Mott & Davis, 1986).

Ability to control parasitic diseases in water schemes depends on the health service infrastructure, which varies from country to country in terms of managerial capacity and operational efficiency. Some countries can mobilize a large cadre of trained public health workers to deal with epidemics but still have to confront the dilemma of vertical efficiency versus lack of coordination with the general health services as they strive to maintain short-term achievements and monitor changes in the epidemiological patterns of the diseases.

In water development schemes there is a general lack of means of identifying the priority parasitic diseases that might be exacerbated following project completion. On the other hand, excellent health services and control programmes may provide adequate medical care and prevent parasitic diseases among workers during construction.

During the construction of the dam at Kainji, Nigeria, *Simulium* and mosquito habitats were controlled within a 50-km radius by drainage and systematic pesticide application. A 150-bed hospital, good housing, household toilets, piped water and recreational facilities were provided for the labour force located at New Bussa (Adekolu-John, 1979a). However, after completion of the project the health care services, vector control programme, and social and sanitation services were not maintained and have irreversibly deteriorated (Adekolu-John, 1979b). A major reason for this was a management decision giving direct budget allocations to the energy-generating authority rather than to the health-promoting infrastructure and services. Moreover, no systematic surveillance or monitoring mechanism was established and neither human nor financial resources were allocated for future interventions. Similar circumstances have arisen elsewhere in Africa.

In the relatively few countries where there are control programmes under ministries of health, activities are directed at controlling malaria and, possibly, schistosomiasis, but not lymphatic filariasis. Onchocerciasis control in West Africa has been the responsibility of the WHO Onchocerciasis Control Programme since 1974. The disease has been successfully controlled in seven countries and the Programme is now being extended into four others. Occasional surveillance of dams and irrigation systems is part of the Programme's activities.

All these control programmes are classified as (1) single disease or vertical and (2) multiple disease or integrated. Current public health terminology refers to vertical and horizontal control, the latter using the primary health care approach. Vertical control involves specialized personnel who, administratively and operationally, act almost independently of the general health care delivery system of dispensaries and hospitals (Liese et al., 1991). Usually, vertical control groups are concerned with only one disease; vector control is performed by applying insecticides or molluscicides, and diagnosis and treatment are carried out.

The history of these operational structures is usually bound up with the colonial era and implicit in them is the goal of eradication. Their past achievements are undisputed, but today, the economic constraints on parasitic disease control in developing countries are overwhelming. One effect has been to modify the implicit objectives. The goal of reducing the effects of disease rather than that of total elimination is now considered feasible and realistic in the development context. This objective can be achieved and maintained by utilizing the health services already in place and training the general health staff in simple measures of control.

Experiences in vertical control programmes

Most health services have a long tradition of maintaining specialized parasitic disease control organizations. Malaria eradication programmes were active in all endemic countries in the 1950s and 1960s, but have since decreased in importance and scope. In the smaller number of countries where schistosomiasis is a national priority, specialized control programmes are in force. The WHO Onchocerciasis Control Programme is highly successful in 11 West African countries; as well as conducting control activities it maintains surveillance of dams. Sleeping sickness or African trypanosomiasis has traditionally been controlled by relatively independent mobile teams, although it is not usually associated with water resources development (Agadzi, 1986).

Schistosomiasis

The general features of schistosomiasis control programmes in some water development schemes are shown in Table 12. The largest such programmes are in Egypt and the Philippines. The financial and human resources in these projects are substantial and linked with agricultural financing from multilateral sources. In Egypt, schistosomiasis control accounted for 8% of the budgeted cost of all government health services in 1984 (Webbe & El-Hak, 1990).

Egypt

Aswan High Dam
Schistosomiasis is the major concern of the Ministry of Health. Control activities focus on the 5000 fishermen and their families residing on the islands or along the shore, and on labourers in adjacent agricultural projects. The intermediate snail hosts of *S. haematobium* are abundant on the islands and the lake shore. In 1980 the prevalence of the disease ranged from 9% in Abu Simbel to 75% in Forkondi. Control measures conducted by the Department of Endemic Diseases of the Ministry of Health and the rural health units include: (1) systematic snail sampling at fishermen's settlements and near agricultural developments, followed by focal application of molluscicides; (2) examination of fishermen for the presence of disease, and (3) treatment with the antischistosomal drug, praziquantel, of infected people seeking admission to the lake area from the north, in what is termed "gateway screening". Prevalence is still high, partly because of migration and inadequate sanitation and water supplies.

Upper and Middle Egypt
A control project was established in Upper and Middle Egypt in 1976–77 with loans from the International Bank for Reconstruction and Development. It covers an area of 400 000 ha between Assiut and Dairut (Webbe & El-Hak, 1990). The strategy for control of *S. haematobium* infection in three phases was based on area-wide molluscicide application with selective chemotherapy, using metrifonate initially and praziquantel after 1988. About 70% of the budget was allocated for molluscicide treatments and 30% for chemotherapy. Although the expenditure is considerable, the results up to 1988 were encouraging: the overall prevalence of urinary schistosomiasis dropped from 29.4% to 3.8% in fixed-sample cohort

Table 12. General features of schistosomiasis control programmes in water development schemes

Country	Location	Programme	Population covered	Evaluation	Remarks
Egypt	WHO Research and Training Project, Bahara Governorate	Molluscicide application only	Villages at project site		Started 1961, terminated 1973
	Lake Nasser	Chemotherapy only	7000	Prevalence reduced	Started 1974 and continuing
	Upper Egypt	Molluscicide application and chemotherapy	5 200 000	Prevalence reduced	Started 1980 and continuing
	Middle Egypt	Molluscicide application and chemotherapy	4 200 000	Prevalence reduced	Started 1977 and continuing
	Fayoum	Molluscicide application and chemotherapy	1 163 000	Prevalence reduced	Started 1969 and continuing
	Giza	Molluscicide application and chemotherapy	3 200 000	Prevalence reduced	Started 1983 and continuing
Ghana	WHO inter-regional hydroelectric project	Trials on chemotherapy; molluscicide application; provision of bore holes	Villages at project sites	Prevalence and intensity of infection reduced	Terminated 1981
Islamic Republic of Iran	Khuzestan	Chemotherapy, molluscicide application and engineering	Whole region	Prevalence reduced	Started 1960 and continuing
Jordan	Dam sites	Treatment and molluscicide application	Dam area	No new cases found	Started recently

Madagascar	Two districts of Mahajanga Province	Chemotherapy, health education and water supplies	153 000	Prevalence reduced	Started recently and continuing
Malawi	Several districts	Treatment, health education and sanitation	Villages in project area	Prevalence reduced	Started 1980 and continuing
Mali	National programme	Chemotherapy, health education, water supply and focal molluscicide application	100 villages	Prevalence reduced	Started 1978 and continuing
Saudi Arabia	Scattered reservoirs	Chemotherapy and molluscicide application	Villages around reservoirs	Cases reduced	Started recently
Sudan	El Girba Irrigation Scheme, Blue Nile Health Project	Village planning with essential health and social services, e.g., schools, health centres, piped water, latrines	Settled population (50 000)	10% prevalence sustained	Started 1976 and continuing

villages between 1977 and 1988, and from 16.1% to 4.6% in a 10% household sample between 1979 and 1988 (Webbe & El-Hak, 1990).

Similar reductions occurred in the 800 000-ha irrigated area of Upper Egypt between Aswan and Assiut: the overall prevalence of urinary schistosomiasis dropped from 25.8% to 7.7% in fixed-sample cohort villages between 1980 and 1988, and from 23.6% to 7.3% in a 10% household sample between 1981 and 1988 (Webbe & El-Hak, 1990).

Chemotherapy has an increasing role in Middle and Upper Egypt. Between 1974 and 1984 in Middle Egypt, for example, measures against snails accounted for nearly 70% of the cost of control, half of which went on purchase of molluscicide with hard currency (Egypt, 1987). In 1988 snail control took up 40% of the budget (Webbe & El-Hak, 1990). This tendency has important strategic implications in the prevention and control of schistosomiasis. Chemotherapy has the leading operational role in areas of high risk and is effective in reducing both the prevalence and the severity of the disease.

Nile Delta

The current control strategy is seen in a project initiated in 1990 in the Governorates of Minufiya, Gharbiya and Kafr el Sheikh, with a loan from the African Development Bank. The main objective is to control *S. mansoni*, while the control of *S. haematobium* is also sought, by molluscicide application and chemotherapy; 70% of the budget will go to chemotherapy and 30% to snail control. Selective molluscicide application will be used in the second year after selective chemotherapy with praziquantel. Epidemiological data will provide criteria for molluscicide usage. No molluscicide will be used in villages where the prevalence of *S. mansoni* is less than 20%.

Health education programmes in schools have been intensified to reduce water contact. Television spots indicating the link between behaviour and the acquisition and spread of schistosomiasis, and drawing attention to the availability of safe effective treatment, are regularly shown at peak viewing times.

Ghana

The 80 000 people displaced by the creation of Lake Volta were offered accommodation in 52 new townships built at various distances from it (Graham, 1986). A slightly larger number, mainly fishing families from the lagoons lying along the lower part of the Volta River and from its delta, were attracted to the lake by the rich harvests in the early years of impoundment. They settled along the shore, creating about 1000 new communities, many of which were accessible only by boat.

The formation of Lake Volta in 1964 created an ideal environment for *Bulinus truncatus rohlfsi* the intermediate snail host of urinary schistosomiasis, resulting in an explosive increase in transmission in most communities along the lake (Paperna, 1969). A WHO/UNDP schistosomiasis project was established along a 60-km stretch on the Pawnpawn branch of Lake Volta in 1971 to study the epidemiology and control of the disease. Snail control with molluscicides at human/water contact sites, and selective chemotherapy with metrifonate, were started in 1975.

Financial support from the United Nations Development Programme ended in 1978 and, from 1979 to 1981, the project was mainly supported by WHO (Chu et al., 1981). By the end of the six-year intervention in 1981, prevalence had been reduced from 73.4% to 36.8%, and egg concentration in urine had declined from 47.3 to 13.7 eggs per 5 ml of urine (K. Y. Chu, personal communication, 1981).

Indonesia

Although only about 10 000 people are at risk of schistosomiasis due to *S. japonicum* in the Lindu, Napu and Besoa Valleys, an intensive control programme has been in force since 1981. Mass examination and the treatment of all infected persons with praziquantel have taken place annually, together with the application of molluscicides at 160 transmission sites. Community water supplies and latrines have been provided. The prevalence of the disease in Lindu Valley was reduced from 37.5% in 1972 to 17% in 1981 and to 1.5% in 1988; in Napu Valley the prevalence was 43% in 1972, 37% in 1981, and 2.8% in 1989 (Gani & Rivany, 1989; Isrin, 1989). Infection rates remain high in dogs, pigs and other domestic animals, as well as in wild mammalian reservoirs: 31.6% and 20% respectively in Napu Valley in 1989. The zoonotic cycle threatens to maintain transmission to people.

The cost of the attempt to eradicate schistosomiasis has been high. Mass screening and treatment will probably have to continue indefinitely since the risk of reinfection remains. There is a plan to build a dam on the Gumbasa River at the lake outlet and a feasibility study is to be made. Thousands of workers would be needed and there would be a risk of an explosive increase in the incidence of schistosomiasis during the construction period (Gani & Rivany, 1989). Furthermore, the transmigration programme bringing new residents from Java has continued since 1978. In the village of Owo in Lindu Valley, 50% of the 500 transmigrants became infected within a year after arrival. The transmigrants in the village of Bamba became infected and subsequently left the area (Gani & Rivany, 1989).

Islamic Republic of Iran

The Dez Dam was completed in 1963 in an area where urinary schisto-somiasis was known to be endemic (Oomen et al., 1988). A new system of concrete-lined canals parallel with existing earth canals was completed in 1965 to irrigate 22 000 ha of land. The old irrigation canals then acted as drains and have played an important role in the transmission of urinary schistosomiasis (Chu et al., 1968). A schistosomiasis project was estab-lished in early 1960 with support from WHO and the Near East Founda-tion in the USA. Chemotherapy and molluscicide application have been used to control the disease. In addition a swamp was drained and filled to reduce the numbers of snail habitats and mosquito breeding places.

These integrated control measures have reduced the prevalence and intensity of infection, despite extension of the irrigation system (Arfaa et al., 1970). The average prevalence in the area of endemicity dropped to 8.1% in 1970 and to 0.7% in 1979 (Massoud et al., 1982).

Jordan

In 1984 at King Talal Dam and elsewhere, snails were discovered to be transmitting urinary schistosomiasis. Molluscicide application was used to control the snails while infected foreign workers and local inhabitants were successfully treated (Arfaa, 1988a).

Kenya

Both problems and successes in the control of parasitic diseases in water development projects have been reported (Chowdhury, 1975, 1979; Jordan, 1985; Waiyaki, 1987). The Yala Swamp, covering 16 000 ha, is 80 km from Kisumu on the shores of Lake Victoria. A pilot irrigation scheme covering 212 ha, supported by the United Nations Development Programme and the Food and Agriculture Organization of the United Nations became operational in 1969 in Bunyala (Chowdhury, 1975, 1979). The initial prevalences of *S. mansoni* and *S. haematobium* infection were 17.5% and 6.5% respectively (Sanecki & Diamant, 1967). Only *Bulinus africanus* was found in the irrigation system itself. Molluscicide applications with trifenmorph were too infrequent and the dose was too low. *Biomphalaria pfeifferi, Bulinus truncatus* and *Bulinus ugandae* were dis-covered in 1972 while molluscicide application had been temporarily suspended. The concentration of molluscicide and application frequency were increased over the next four years, during which time all snail habitats were controlled. No recent data are available.

In the Hola Irrigation Scheme, prevalence increased from a high baseline in an area of endemicity. Prevalence remains high despite a sophisticated environmental sanitation programme and systematic molluscicide application.

The Mwea Irrigation Scheme is another area where prevalence has increased dramatically. However, snail surveillance and molluscicide application, although not performed regularly, have kept snail populations down. In the 35 villages most of the 3000 plot-holders and their families draw water from the river. Diagnosis and treatment are now available in the health facilities attached to the scheme. It appears that the transmission of schistosomiasis in surrounding villages contributes to the maintenance of the disease in the scheme.

The Ahero Irrigation Scheme has maintained minimal molluscicide application in an area where the prevalence of intestinal schistosomiasis and populations of *Biomphalaria* have always been low. Transmission probably occurs more in the vicinity of nearby rivers than in the irrigation system itself.

The Perkerra Irrigation Scheme of 415 ha, with a potential coverage of 3500 ha, has never been an area of high endemicity and transmission has been low, although the intermediate snail hosts for both urinary and intestinal schistosomiasis are present.

In the most recent and largest of the National Irrigation Board's schemes, the Bura Irrigation Scheme covering 6700 ha, located north of the Hola scheme, snail populations have been maintained at low levels by the systematic application of niclosamide. Within the project area, the prevalence of urinary schistosomiasis among schoolchildren is around 20%. However, in surrounding villages the prevalence reaches over 60% (Waiyaki, 1987).

Madagascar

In two districts of Mahajanga Province, where agricultural development and irrigation programmes are in progress, the transmission of *S. haematobium* constitutes a major health problem. The programme intervention area comprises the districts of Marovoay and Port Berge, which have a population of 153 000. The goal is to reduce the prevalence of schistosomiasis to levels that can be managed by the local rural health services.

Strategies for active intervention rely primarily on mass chemotherapy with praziquantel but also include health education and a limited programme to improve village water supplies. The type of mass chemotherapy provided in the villages depends on the prevalence of *S. haematobium* found during baseline sample surveys. If it is over 50%, all inhabitants are treated; if it is between 20% and 50% all are examined but only those found to be infected are treated; and if it is under 20%, only those found positive in a sample are treated.

75

Two years after a single intervention, prevalence in these villages dropped to below 16% (Brinkmann et al., 1989).

Malawi

On undertaking agricultural development projects in the early 1970s the Ministry of Agriculture introduced limited control programmes against the snail intermediate hosts of S. mansoni and S. haematobium. During 1980–86, the Federal Republic of Germany assisted schistosomiasis control in several districts of Malawi. Since 1986, schistosomiasis control has been extended.

The goal of the programme is to lower the prevalence of heavy infections to less than 5% in children and to less than 2% in adults. A heavy infection is defined as the excretion of more than 50 eggs per 10 ml of urine for S. haematobium or more than 100 eggs per g of faeces for S. mansoni.

Treatment, health education and sanitation are used to control the disease. So far, significant reductions in general prevalence and intensity of infection have been achieved in a substantial number of settlements in pilot areas. It is too early to report results for the country as a whole (Brinkmann et al., 1989).

Mali

Schistosomiasis is one of the most important health problems associated with man-made lakes and irrigated areas in Mali. S. haematobium, S. mansoni and S. intercalatum are present. With assistance from the Federal Republic of Germany, control activities were started in Bandiagara during 1978. In 1982 a national programme of schistosomiasis control was created as part of a 10-year plan for the development of health services.

The main strategy for schistosomiasis control consists of a combination of chemotherapy, health education, and the provision of clean water. Focal snail control is limited to important transmission sites.

More than 100 villages with a total population of about 75 000 have been covered by control operations in the intervention areas, resulting in a reduction in prevalence of about 50%. About 80% of the goals set for the intervention phase have been reached in the rural areas (Brinkmann et al., 1989).

Philippines

Water resources development is a national priority in the Philippines. In the 1983–87 five-year development plan, irrigation alone accounted for 27.9% of the total investment of US$ 4.34 thousand million. The development of water resources for irrigation is coordinated by the National

Irrigation Administration, a government-owned corporation since 1964. In 1984 no less than 31 irrigation projects were being implemented with foreign support, covering the rehabilitation of 166 000 ha and the new development of 450 000 ha. At that time 1.4 million ha were being irrigated, which represented 44% of the country's irrigable land (Tech, 1984).

The National Irrigation System Improvement Project in Leyte began in 1979 with loan assistance from the World Bank. The strategy included

— case-finding and treatment of all infected persons;
— provision of safe water supplies and water-sealed toilets;
— snail control through drainage of waterlogged areas;
— construction of footbridges;
— public health education.

The prevalence of schistosomiasis in the population at risk, about 200 000 people, fell from 23.6% in 1979 to 9.3% in 1985.

Of the budget for the schistosomiasis control component of the programme, 74.5% was spent on drainage, 17.8% on case-finding, treatment and health education, and 7.6% on toilets, handpumps and footbridges.

Blas (1989) estimated that 19.2 days of work per annum were gained by individuals who were treated. On this basis the economic benefit to Leyte alone, assuming that half the treated population earned a minimum wage, would be US$ 1 million. For the whole country the figure would be over US$ 8 million.

Saudi Arabia

Schistosomiasis has spread in parts of Saudi Arabia as a result of water development. The primary health care system of peripheral dispensaries and health clinics has been the chief means of undertaking and sustaining control. Systematic case-finding on a large scale and treatment have been performed by the staff of the clinics. Where feasible, molluscicides have been applied in places of frequent water contact and high densities of snail intermediate hosts.

A large reservoir created during the past decade near Medina became highly infested with *Biomphalaria arabica*, but molluscicide applications have successfully prevented any extension of transmission.

In Al Baha Region, 18 of 21 reservoirs created in recent years have become densely populated with *Biomphalaria arabica* and *Bulinus truncatus*, allowing the transmission of *S. mansoni* to occur in some nearby villages. Urinary schistosomiasis, however, is not increasing because of the resistance of the snails to infection. The primary health care system is now responsible for case-finding and treatment, and prevalence continues to fall.

Another large dam in the Najran Region at the Yemen border was infested with *Bu. beccarii*, the main host of urinary schistosomiasis in Saudi Arabia, resulting in increased prevalences of infection in communities downstream. The focal use of molluscicides at points of water contact, and the diagnosis and treatment of individual cases have been successful (Arfaa, 1988b).

Swaziland

In the irrigated estates of the Commonwealth Development Corporation, where the prevalence of schistosomiasis was generally high, several interventions were effective. Differences in the prevalence of schistosomiasis were generally related to the presence or condition of piped water supplies, communal toilets, and laundry facilities. It was noted that water contact and transmission continued unless access to transmission sites was prevented by fences and bridges and snail control was sustained. Most importantly, a management policy of maintaining a stable work force with reduced seasonal labour improved the efficiency of disease control (Logan, 1983).

Logan (1983) reported that the prevalence of schistosomiasis on three irrigated estates was lower than in nearby estates in the Transvaal (South Africa). He attributed this to the presence of adequate domestic water supplies, communal toilets, laundry facilities, and agricultural and irrigation practices of a high standard, including the use of concrete-lined canals, subsoil drainage, and appropriately increased water flow rates in lined or realigned canals. Chaine (1984) observed that, although on irrigated estates there was a raised risk of exposure to schistosomiasis because of the creation of potential transmission sites, there were also better living conditions that promoted control.

Zimbabwe

The Hippo Valley/Triangle Estates irrigation area includes 54 adjacent farms bounded by the Mtilikwe, Chiredzi and Lundi Rivers. Within the 380-km² area under control there are 285 km² of irrigated land, 307 storage dams with a total capacity of 4.5 million m³, over 600 km of lined canals and about 1500 km of drains and streams. The population is unstable, varying between 75 000 and 100 000, of whom 20 500 are employees of the Estates.

Various schemes of molluscicide application have been successfully used since 1969. The prevalence of *S. mansoni* among schoolchildren, which was above 70% at the outset, was kept below 30% from 1977 until 1980. The prevalence of *S. haematobium* was relatively unchanged at around 40% throughout this period (Evans, 1983).

In the smallholding irrigation schemes at Mushandike in south-east Zimbabwe, particular attention was given to the location of settlements and the provision of safe water supplies and sanitation (Chandiwana et al., 1988). In the irrigation system all secondary and tertiary canals were lined with concrete. The designs of the sluice gates, weirs and off-takes diminished any damming effect. Snail populations were reduced by measures such as the regular drying out of the canals, the fluctuation of water levels in reservoirs, routine cleaning, the removal of debris and vegetation, and the prevention of seepage. Water usage was maximized by growing particular crops at particular times—maize and cotton between November and March, and wheat and vegetables between June and August.

Villages were located as far as possible, but not more than 1 km from the fields, as in the Sudan (Blue Nile Health Project, 1985). Bore holes were fitted with handpumps, and washing slabs were located nearby. Technical support was available to ensure the proper construction of latrines, and cement was provided free as an incentive.

In two of these schemes the effect of chemotherapy was dramatic between April 1986 and August 1987, lowering the prevalence of urinary schistosomiasis from 18.7% to 8.8% and from 17.7% to 3.2%; the prevalence of *S. mansoni* was reduced from 3.9% to 0.7% and from 2.6% to 0% in the same localities. On the other hand, in a community where the irrigation management approach was not implemented and only treatment was given, the prevalence of *S. haematobium* declined from 34.8% to 24.2% and that of *S. mansoni* increased slightly from 5.4% to 6.9%.

This experience has confirmed that engineering and environmental measures that are beneficial to agricultural production and the quality of life significantly enhance the effect of chemotherapy.

Malaria

Malaria is the most widespread parasitic disease associated with water resources projects. Its prevalence and rates of morbidity and mortality are highest in Asia and Africa. In many African countries there is virtually no control of malaria.

China

The world's largest area of irrigated rice fields is in China. Residual indoor spraying of walls of dwellings has not been effective in controlling malaria transmission. In 1978, environmental management was considered to be one of the most important control approaches and the intermittent or wet irrigation method was found to be highly effective (Lu, 1984). Wet irrigation is practised in Hunan Province and, in one trial, it reduced the population of *A. sinensis* by 53–55% and that of *C. tritaeniorhyncus* by 55–70% (Lu, 1984).

India

In Mysore, Rao (1945) reported an increase in the proportion of palpable spleens from 15% to 50% and a twentyfold rise in deaths due to malaria following the opening of the Visvesvaraya Canal. Fortunately, continuously applied antimalarial measures have reduced the level of infection.

Intermittent irrigation of rice fields to control malaria was first studied in southern India (Russell et al., 1940). In 1941 land drainage, canal improvement and the relocation of 200 villages to well protected sites preceded the commissioning of an irrigation project. Biological control was introduced in ten villages. This strategy eliminated malaria during the four-year experimental period. However, in spite of the success achieved, it has not been followed up in most rice-growing areas because of the technical problems involved (Bang & Pant, 1983).

Indonesia

In the heavily populated Central Java Province, irrigated rice fields account for about 90% of the total cultivated land and malaria is endemic. Indoor residual spraying has been carried out regularly since 1952 (Bang, 1988). Malaria control through intermittent irrigation, tested with the help of financial support from WHO, has reduced the overall population densities of mosquitos and other pests. Currently an integrated programme is in place, involving the use of larvivorous fish, intermittent irrigation, and the growing of rice on slopes to permit good drainage. These measures have reduced the proportion of palpable spleens from 16.5% in 1929 to 0.2% in 1984 (Bang, 1988).

Transmigration of people between islands of the Indonesian archipelago is strongly associated with disease outbreaks, especially of malaria and filariasis around water projects (Abisudjak & Kotanegara, 1989).

Nigeria

A programme for the control of mosquitos and blackfly (*Simulium*) based on the use of DDT larvicide within a radius of 50 km of Kainji Dam, was operational from 1961 until recently (Adekolu-John, 1983). With the creation of Jebba Lake in 1984 the breeding sites below the Kainji Dam were eliminated. Vector control activities continue sporadically in neighbouring streams although Waddy (1972) reported low parasitaemia rates among children in New Bussa, a town in the control area.

Lymphatic filariasis

Lymphatic filariasis is endemic in Africa, but the scale of the public health problem is greatest in the Pacific area, China, India and Indonesia, where more than two-thirds of the world's infected population reside (WHO, 1992a). Extensive dam-building for irrigation, especially of rice, has been observed to increase vector populations in Africa and Indonesia (Hunter, 1992). Separate control measures against lymphatic filariasis are not known to exist anywhere in water resources development schemes, but China, India and Indonesia have established mosquito control measures in some of their schemes. It would appear that such measures are partially effective against lymphatic filariasis.

Neither lymphatic filariasis nor Japanese encephalitis has been used as an index to evaluate vector control measures in water development schemes.

An integrated programme: the Blue Nile Health Project

With the support of WHO, the Blue Nile Health Project was established in 1979 to control malaria, schistosomiasis and diarrhoea in irrigated areas through a multisectoral, comprehensive approach. The project includes the Gezira Irrigation Scheme, the Managil Extension between the Blue Nile and the White Nile, and the new Rahad Scheme. The goal is to keep malaria prevalence at 2% or below, to reduce schistosomiasis prevalence from the 1979 level of 50% to 10%, and to reduce mortality due to diarrhoeal diseases (Blue Nile Health Project, 1985; Fenwick, 1989). The strategy includes:

- health education and community participation;
- provision of domestic water supplies and improvement of sanitation;
- the use of residual insecticides and larvicides for the control of mosquitos, and focal chemical control of intermediate snail hosts of schistosomiasis, both intestinal and urinary;
- chemotherapy for malaria and schistosomiasis;
- the use of oral rehydration salts for the treatment of diarrhoea.

Vector control and chemotherapy have been effective in maintaining a low level of malarial parasitaemia in the project area. Routine schistosomiasis control measures reduced prevalence in the special study zone and in the Gezira-Managil zone to 10.2% and 15.5% respectively in 1988. However, in the Rahad area the prevalence of schistosomiasis among schoolchildren increased from 13.2% in 1987 to 18.7% in 1988. Most of the infections were imported.

Malaria was not a major public health problem in Gezira-Managil between 1930 and 1950. Control depended on larval treatment with Paris green and diesel oil applied by the tenant farmers. Adherence to water management practices was required by local legislation. The first residual insecticide, BHC, was introduced in 1950. The mosquito population density was reduced and, by 1965, the parasitaemia rate was as low as 1.9%. Environmental and anti-larval measures were subsequently relaxed. Resistance to BHC appeared in the mosquito population in 1965 and resistance to its replacement, DDT, was widespread by 1970. Between 1970 and 1975, anti-larval measures were re-established but were no longer effective because agricultural intensification had brought about continuous, rather than seasonal, malaria transmission. The prevalence of malaria reached 22.8%, but by 1982 intensive water control and the use of malathion and fenitrothion reduced it to 0.95%. In Gezira the overall prevalence in 1988 was 5.1% while in specially monitored villages it was 0.49%. It is considered by the management of the Blue Nile Health Project that malaria is now under control. Clearly, however, for both schistosomiasis and malaria, constant vigilance is needed (Amin, 1977; Daffalla et al., 1988).

Factors militating against prevention and control

While the above examples may not be universally applicable, they all confirm that the present general paucity of action is unjustifiable. Parasitic diseases are an avoidable risk in water resources projects, and their exacerbation is but one indication of inadequate provision for health in the development strategy. The constraints are multiple. The underlying poverty, the exploitation of labour, especially child labour, and the high population growth rates in development areas driven by macroeconomic objectives, all militate against the prevention and control of disease and the promotion of health.

National level

In the developing countries, parasitic diseases are tolerated by people to a remarkable degree. History and tradition have much to do with this. An improved quality of life does not necessarily mean an absence of parasitic disease as far as the people are concerned. Even where the prevalence of parasitic disease is increasing rapidly the political reaction time is relatively slow. The issues for central government include the following.

- The greatest requirement for control measures arises in countries undergoing rapid development. African countries with high disease rates are in critical need. Decisions are usually taken on an impromptu basis, without consideration for other matters that might be important. Policy-makers are not aware of the benefits of and the need for health promotion and disease control, or of the need to include them from the beginning in plans for water resources development. Disease control appears, if at all, after construction has finished.

- At the centre there is a failure to appreciate that health problems in water developments are ecological in character and that long-term solutions require broad participation and the integration of many sectoral inputs. Poor national coordination and integration hinder disease control.

- Except in epidemic situations resulting in death or disability, health officials have not been able to demonstrate the adverse effects of disease on capital projects in economic terms.

- Donor agencies have a negative or dissociative attitude to health matters in project developments. This means that external support is very weak if recipient countries wish to fund health and control programmes in connection with water resources development.

- Ministries of health have not played their roles effectively as custodians of health in major development projects. They are usually neither assertive nor confrontational in defining the health risks associated with projects, and fail to provide technical options or to identify intersectoral input for the prevention and control of parasitic diseases. They have not rallied political support that might ensure the consideration of health risks in project development. Thus they do not fulfil a leadership role in intersectoral communication.

- Political vision is lacking: it is assumed that the price of development has to be paid in terms of disease. The costs of disease are considered to be less than the potential economic benefits. The depth of ignorance in the political sector on the feasibility and simplicity of mitigating negative health effects should be addressed by the health sector.

- Although adequate legislation may require preliminary environmental and health risk assessment in a proposed water resources project, in practice, especially in developing countries, a pro forma document is likely to be prepared to fulfil the legal requirements, without requiring the donor or contractor to prevent or mitigate potential risks.

Local level

The constraints at the field level are a reflection of the lack of orientation and priority at the national level. The people themselves are the first to be affected and the last to be addressed.

- Control programmes are often oriented to only one disease and are centrally managed, so that communities, let alone agencies participating independently in the development process, have no linkage with the activities undertaken, and consequently the best possible use of resources is not achieved.
- Trained personnel are often not available locally to investigate, plan and evaluate control programmes.
- Resources for maintenance and replacement continue to diminish in response to economic recession.
- Community participation through women's groups, local political groups, and nongovernmental organizations is rarely harmonized with control activities.
- Databases on health and disease emanating directly and indirectly from water resources developments are often inadequate. Health effects need to be documented at local level and analysed, usually at the central level, in order to assess the implications for planning and policy development. Ultimately, the quality of planning and implementation of control programmes is strongly influenced by the quality and extent of data on parasitic diseases.

International level

The international development community remains relatively insensitive to the risks of parasitic diseases in water resources projects. WHO is attempting to persuade international funding agencies and national governments to accept responsibility for the health implications of this kind of development. It is necessary to provide reliable data on parasitic diseases, to encourage WHO collaborating centres and national experts to participate in feasibility and planning studies, and to include water resources development in all plans of action for the control of filariasis, malaria and schistosomiasis. The highly successful Onchocerciasis Control Programme in West Africa (WHO, 1991) has used proven methods of vector control, and ivermectin has enhanced the feasibility of combating the disease. WHO can provide specific technical advice on the prevention and control of these parasitic diseases which is adaptable to water re-sources projects.

Significantly, WHO has given special attention to involving health authorities in the discussion of development policy. A symposium held in Bangalore (WHO Regional Office for South-East Asia, 1989) represented the first attempt to strengthen the negotiating skills of ministries of health and other relevant sectors with a view to defending the health status of people in development projects.

Feasible intervention approaches

Development of essential services and infrastructure is the best long-term investment for disease control in water resources projects. Their absence or inefficiency is often the result of inadequate planning and coordination, beginning with preliminary feasibility studies. Numerous checklists have been prepared so that the risks of waterborne diseases will be recognized early. This approach has been designed by specialists working directly on the diseases, and consequently the communication of the message and the incorporation of preventive measures into actual interventions may not always be very efficient.

Among the essential services, general health care through a dispensary and hospital system is fundamental for the implementation and mainten-ance of disease control. The investment in basic health services as part of a project plan is likely to have a greater long-term effect than costly independent disease-specific control.

At the other end of the spectrum the tradition of specialized control agencies has been encouraged by the international donor community. These agencies are technically effective and may even be efficient. How-ever, the question of sustainability arises. With the current means of controlling parasitic diseases it is short-sighted and inefficient not to make provision for maintaining control through the general health services. Concentrated and labour-intensive action is necessary by trained pro-fessional staff in the early phase of any control activities. Their role, however, becomes more and more managerial and supervisory as control targets are achieved.

Population groups at risk

Population groups that are likely to be at risk of health problems associ-ated with water development schemes include settled or host populations, resettled populations, migrant labourers and fishermen, and tourists. Workers on a project site could also be at high risk by virtue of their constant exposure to the water resource. The planning of disease control programmes in water resources development schemes requires the identification of different population groups according to their proximity to and association with water. Some people, including settled and resettled populations, itinerant labourers, and migrants, may have relatively infrequent contact with water, while fishermen, irrigation farmers and workers engaged in project operations and maintenance are virtually in continuous contact with water.

Integrated control

The technical details behind the strategies for the control of parasitic diseases in water resources projects are indicated in WHO documents. Expert committees prepare technical guidelines for control which are conceptually up to date and provide the latest information on pesticides, drugs and equipment (WHO, 1985, 1986b, 1986c, 1987a, 1990, 1992a, 1993; WHO/UNEP, 1990). Those engaged in the development process should consult these documents which outline feasible approaches for all situations, even where resources are limited.

Vertical programmes that achieved early success in many countries have gradually fallen out of favour because of vector resistance to pesticides, parasite resistance to drugs, difficulties in the management of the environment, and problems in the control of vectors and intermediate hosts by water management. It is important to note that the maintenance of the infrastructure of vertical programmes becomes increasingly expensive in the face of global economic recession. However, as previously noted, an integrated comprehensive control strategy in line with the philosophy of primary health care was recently successful in the Sudan against schistosomiasis, malaria and diarrhoea (Amin, 1977; Daffalla et al., 1988). This strategy has been endorsed by management as yielding a reasonable return on investment in the Gezira (Fadl, 1990), and should be considered for wider adoption in water resources development. The principal features of a comprehensive, integrated control strategy are as follows.

- A well executed housing programme, equitable house compensation policy, and appropriate agricultural resettlement programme. Such a programme was implemented in the Kpong Resettlement Programme in Ghana, and provided essential intersectoral input for control of parasitic diseases (Futa, 1983).

- The provision of domestic water supplies, adequate housing for resettled populations, improved sanitation and village planning. This is the most permanent and significant contribution to health and the quality of life.

- A basic health services infrastructure with planned provision of staff, supervision and a specified role in the monitoring and surveillance of waterborne diseases. Health services in water resources projects should not be viewed as curative enterprises. Their public health role should be defined and the capacity to undertake prevention and control should be adequately supported.

- Health education integrated into health services, schools and community activities. The message in the health education package should be carefully considered and developed with professional input, and evaluated. This is a unique opportunity to influence popular perceptions about water, environment and health.

- Community involvement in health programmes, particularly those concerned with maternal and child health, and community participation in health matters in local government. A sense of personal and collective responsibility for environment- and health-linked issues is growing. The questions of solid waste disposal, pollution and other forms of environmental degradation can be resolved at this level.

- Vector control through the coordinated action of specialized personnel in ministries of health and agencies responsible for public works, roads, construction, irrigation and other forms of environmental modification, e.g., the filling and drainage of unnecessary bodies of water, the fencing of ponds in areas where children play, house spraying, the application of larvicides, and the elimination of breeding sites (Coosemans & Barutwanayo, 1989; Mouchet & Brengues, 1990). Such technical activity has become an exclusive responsibility of specialized personnel. Dialogue with the community, if specifically planned with appropriate messages and instructions, could facilitate the work of vector control and could even contribute directly to the identification and reduction of breeding sites as well as to the use of personal protection.

- Diagnosis and treatment of parasitic diseases, e.g., malaria, schistosomiasis and lymphatic filariasis. The treatment of schistosomiasis has proved cost-effective in tin-mining operations in Zaire (Polderman, 1984). Peripheral laboratory facilities and a drug policy whereby appropriate drugs are made available for the treatment of parasitic diseases can strengthen the delivery system.

- Motivation to produce food crops of high nutrient value. This can be promoted as part of the education programme, in coordination with agricultural extension workers.

Within the health care systems of water resources projects, other problems can be tackled:

— immunization against common communicable diseases, including yellow fever, Japanese encephalitis, cerebrospinal meningitis and childhood diseases;
— limitation of population growth through family planning;
— provision of essential drugs;
— establishment of effective emergency services with ambulance-supported referral;
— training of village health workers and microscopists.

This strategy is recommended for implementation in villages and settlements where there is a high frequency of contact with the water of reservoirs, irrigated areas and drainage channels.

Environmental control of snails and mosquitos

A wide range of engineering techniques have been advocated for the control of intermediate hosts of parasitic diseases (Blas, 1976; Bolton, 1988; Cairncross & Feachem, 1983; Lanoix, 1958; Pike, 1987; Oomen et al., 1990).

Design and construction of canals
- Canal beds should be properly elevated to prevent formation of pools of stagnant water.
- Canals should be lined with concrete, or with cement blocks and polyethylene, to prevent silt deposition, the formation of shallow sunlit pools, and overflowing.
- Construction should be properly supervised to ensure good workmanship and the use of materials of high quality.
- Sprinkler and trickle irrigation should replace the older methods.

Operation and maintenance
- Water management practices inherent in optimal agricultural production, if maintained, contribute to vector control.
- Canals, reservoirs and fish ponds should be periodically cleared of weeds, and forestry management applied close to reservoirs and canals.

Environmental modification
- Unnecessary bodies of water should be filled and drained.
- Bridges should be built where fording is common.
- Adequate water supplies, latrines and bathing facilities should be provided.
- Health education on the transmission of waterborne diseases should be given, with emphasis on preventive and control measures.

In 1981, attention was focused by WHO, FAO and UNEP on environmental management for the control of vectorborne diseases. During the same year a Panel of Experts on Environmental Management for Vector Control was established, with the objective of creating an institutional framework for interagency and intersectoral collaboration for health, water and land development and for protection of the environment. The Panel promotes disease forecasting and the extended use of environmental management measures for vector control (Mather & That, 1984; WHO/FAO/UNEP, 1986, 1987a; Birley, 1989; Tiffen, 1989).

Epidemiological evaluation, monitoring and surveillance

In water resources schemes it is fundamental to institute surveillance based on the health care delivery system. If diagnosis and treatment of parasitic diseases are available, then the data obtained should be reported systematically and reviewed at higher levels, where operational decisions on specific interventions can be made. In the Amazon Basin, for example, where the intermediate snail host is present and infectious human carriers may be introduced, the examination of parasitological reports may give the first indication of increased transmission. The numbers of cases of malaria may suddenly increase, but monitoring of hospitalizations is retrospective rather than preventive; hence the need for frequent observation and early warning.

Donors and even national planning agencies rely heavily on in-depth, short-term studies or surveys to obtain projections of the risks of parasitic diseases, since there are often few routine reports and analyses of data by national health services. The negotiating position of a ministry of health is strengthened if such data are available internally. On the other hand, if money is scarce, the ministry should be able to prepare a well-conceived plan with a request for external financial support for surveillance. This type of proposal should envisage both short-term and long-term needs: for pre-impoundment analysis, the installation and maintenance of health services, the monitoring of parasitic disease patterns, prevention, and health promotion among all the populations involved.

The assessment of the success of a control strategy requires planned surveillance. Health problems vary from country to country and within individual countries, as do ecosystems and other variables that influence the health situation. Various clinical, parasitological and entomological parameters, previously used in vertical control programmes, have inherent advantages and disadvantages. The indicators selected should be simple and economical to measure, and meet local requirements. The guiding principle is to achieve reductions in disease morbidity and mortality. The follow-up indicators for all population groups are indicated below.

- *Malaria:*
  — prevalence of fever;
  — spleen rate;
  — slide positivity rate.

- *Schistosomiasis:*
  — prevalence of haematuria;
  — prevalence and intensity of eggs in urine and stools.

- *Lymphatic filariasis:*
  — slide positivity rate;
  — prevalence of hydrocele and elephantiasis.

- *Onchocerciasis:*
  — prevalence of microfilariae in skin snips;
  — prevalence of blindness.

Hospital and dispensary records of the incidence of parasitic diseases as a cause of outpatient consultations and admissions reliably indicate the public health impact and serve to support statements on days of work lost and other direct costs of these diseases in water resources projects.

In programmes that include mosquito and snail control the first step is to identify the species involved. Standard procedures should be used to determine the densities of mosquito vector and intermediate snail host populations. Simple surveillance techniques, even if qualitative, are useful for field staff who wish to monitor changes in these populations. Mosquito population densities may be assessed in terms of the number of bites per person per year. Snail population densities are usually recorded as the number of snails found per square metre or after 15 minutes scooping with a sieve. Technical advice is usually available from national services.

Ackers & Smith (1988) have pointed out the validity of measurement of general health indicators, such as birth rate, crude mortality rate and infant mortality rate. Systematic surveillance of rates of diarrhoea, acute respiratory infections, occupational accidents and nutritional status (anaemia, height/weight ratio) are useful for health management in water resources development.

Maintenance of control

Success in the control of parasitic diseases in a water resources project does not simply mean treating all cases. It is important to maintain control, and this requires monitoring at all levels so that changes in vector populations, the migration of infected persons, the use of antiparasitic drugs, and the diagnosis of new cases through laboratory services can be investigated and action taken as required.

When interventions are undertaken, say during a malaria outbreak, vector control and case detection are rightly done by specialized emergency personnel who are organizationally independent of the routine health services. They have no responsibility for training local health workers who are present during the outbreak and who will remain afterwards. These training needs are best met by long-term in-service programmes.

The ministry of health can strengthen its negotiating position by having both a short-term and a long-term perspective on the control of parasitic diseases and by integrating these activities into all health programmes. If this is done, maintenance becomes an established feature rather than a crisis reaction. For long-term success, efforts should be directed towards integrating the health care and disease control programmes of water development projects into national health schemes.

6.

Policy critique of health aspects of water development projects

Why has there been a failure to implement, in a systematic manner, the technical approaches outlined in the preceding chapter? An attempt has to be made to arrive at relevant pragmatic policies, whereby the prevention and control of parasitic diseases becomes an established routine accepted by financiers, planners and managers of water resources projects. In this connection, one of the roles of WHO is to help to create an informed body of opinion leading to demands for the inclusion of adequate health care infrastructures in all future schemes of water impoundment and irrigation (Cooper Weil et al., 1990).

Compartmentalism

Some decades ago it was arguable that those engaged in water development planning were unaware of the possible health consequences of their actions, being uninformed and ecologically naive. Such excuses are no longer acceptable. Much is known and expected, and there is a widespread awareness of the possible ecological effects of water impoundment, including increases in the incidence of parasitic and infectious diseases. Refuge can no longer be taken in narrow sectoral planning compartments because the real world is not segregated in this way.

The problems of river basin development have been repeatedly divided into separate administrative and bureaucratic entities. Past conflicts of interest, gaps in implementation and lapses in responsibility, and the resultant glaring neglect of key health issues, seemingly have no effect on the future execution of projects. Without any presumption of moral superiority, one might feel that it is highly unethical to ignore the health hazards that have been created.

Significant regional and local asymmetries of benefit and risk are typically found in water impoundment schemes involving irrigation and power production. Many people living in towns, participating in the wider national economy, benefit from electricity, salaried employment and other economic advantages, whereas those living near the bodies of water suffer from increased disease and are even worse off than before. Thus social and economic imbalance between different regions is accentuated. Environmental degradation in lake areas contrasts starkly with the improved quality of life elsewhere. To remedy this situation national planning mechanisms should be established with the purpose of reducing regional inequalities through both risk reduction and better spread of benefits.

Economic progress or health?

The apparent interests of water impoundments and irrigation schemes continue to conflict with those of human health. Worthington (1977) admitted that irrigated agriculture and health can be seen as opposed to one another but argued that they could be made complementary. To achieve this is a basic challenge.

How should the argument that disease is an inescapable consequence of progress be regarded? One view is that it is essential to construct many new dams and reservoirs and that environmental and health costs are inevitable and have to be absorbed in order to secure overall benefits (McJunkin, 1975; World Bank/IMF, 1987). However, this is not an either/or situation. Preventive health measures can be introduced into water development projects without impairing their efficiency or their priority objectives for economic development. Moreover, such measures can be expected to increase productive efficiency. In any case, is it econometrically valid to omit future health costs from the debit/credit balance or discount rates? There is clear evidence from the agricultural sector on the impact of malaria and schistosomiasis in large schemes, such as that of the Gezira, where many working days are lost because of illness (Fadl, 1990).

In entering into the intersectoral dialogue, the health sector should recognize that other costs, not internalized in water resources development, may be even less predictable than those of disease because of their latency, such as costs associated with salination, involuntary settlements, cultural property, and biodiversity (Goodland, 1989). All of these factors may also have important long-term negative health effects.

Coordination or sectoralism?

The absence of coordination among administrative bureaucracies such as the ministries responsible for agriculture, irrigation, water supply, electricity, education and health is inefficient and wasteful of national resources. Such institutional separatism usually results in water impoundment schemes being implemented by relatively capital-rich bureaucracies that unintentionally create outbreaks of disease. The cost of managing these is transferred to the capital-poor, underfinanced and infrastructurally weaker health care services. In other words those who create the problem do not share its real costs, whereas, in justice, those who enjoy the scheme's wider benefits should assist those suffering from it; better still, they should prevent the problems from arising in the first place.

Full policy recognition of the essential complementarity of economic development and health would allow coordinated planning for the prevention or minimization of health hazards emerging from water impoundment schemes (Mather & Bos, 1989). This would spread benefits and costs over the nation as a whole. Preventive measures would also promote greater economic production efficiency. Furthermore, as preventive health care is less expensive than curative care, the total real costs to the country would be reduced. Water resources development projects that do not address the essential complementarity of development and health should be challenged by the health sector and the people affected.

The lack of support for control of parasitic diseases is not due solely to sectoral compartmentalization. It is generally agreed among development financing agencies that there has rarely, if ever, been a positive independent proposal by a ministry of health to include a programme for the mitigation and control of parasitic diseases in a water resources project. The usual scenario is that the financing agency approaches the ministry of health to request that a proposal be submitted, but finally has to hire consultants to prepare it since the ministry does not have the necessary staff or available data. On the other hand, how common is it for the financing or lead national agency to invite the ministry of health to participate equitably in the planning process?

Sectoralism hinders internal cooperation in all large organizations, including bilateral assistance agencies. Thus, for example, the USAID bureaucracy that dealt with water resources development in the Mandara Mountains, Cameroon, did not join operationally for planning purposes with the health services administration (J. M. Hunter, personal communication, 1979). Philanthropic institutions are no exception: for instance the Agricultural Sciences Division of the Rockefeller Foundation, which is active in a large irrigation project in Zimbabwe, could not be persuaded by the Foundation's Health Services Division to consider the health hazards of the scheme (K. S. Warren, personal communication, 1989).

Failure to implement international agreements on health protection

There is no lack of memoranda of understanding and agreements on collaboration between international organizations. These agreements take a short-term view and usually lack the executive and administrative support necessary for implementation. Nevertheless, they provide a basis for action and should be revived by countries that would benefit from the coordination of efforts.

The United Nations system has a unique potential for effective co-ordination with Member States. The specialized agencies represent all aspects of development, environment and health of relevance to water resources. The following are some of the formal agreements on this issue.

United Nations Memoranda of Accord

In response to concerns expressed in the United Nations over problems of economic development and health, inter-agency memoranda of under-standing have been established between WHO and the World Bank and between WHO and FAO.

World Bank

A joint memorandum on health activities was signed on behalf of the World Bank and WHO in 1976. It was agreed that the World Bank would assist WHO in analysing and projecting socioeconomic conditions, in assessing national development plans, in planning, implementing and evaluating WHO-assisted projects, in strengthening national health or health-related institutions, and in analysing problems arising from the delivery of health services. It was also agreed that WHO would assist the Bank as required in designing, appraising and monitoring schemes for the delivery of health services, the control of communicable diseases, the planning of health manpower education, the monitoring of health condi-tions, and the conduct of research in the biomedical sciences. Other terms covered field assistance, staff training exchanges, schedules of missions, exchange of information, and annual meetings. It is fair to say that these proposed outcomes have not materialized.

Food and Agriculture Organization of the United Nations

A memorandum of understanding governing collaboration by WHO and FAO in the prevention and control of waterborne diseases associated with water development activities was signed in 1978. The main terms were as follows.

Article 1. Scope of cooperation

The two Organizations were to establish procedures for collaboration in initiating joint action in support of the prevention and control of water-borne diseases. This action was to include the following.

- Reactivation of periodic FAO/WHO project review meetings in order to identify health measures deemed necessary under the objectives of the memorandum of understanding.
- Exchange of information and data on water development projects, in collaboration with UNDP and in the context of the country programme and its periodic reviews.
- Exchange of data on agricultural water development projects funded from sources other than UNDP, to supplement the information referred to in the preceding paragraph.
- Exchange of background information in the form of country briefs (FAO) and country profiles (WHO) in order to maintain up-to-date knowledge on development in agriculture and on health conditions of relevance to the programmes of both Organizations; preparation of summary information sheets for the use of funding agencies, to assist in identifying appropriate action for water development activities.

Article 2. Preparation of guidelines and training

The two Organizations were to cooperate in preparing technical guidelines, checklists and training programmes so that the personnel and institutions responsible for the planning, design, construction and management of water development projects in the Member States would be able to ensure necessary health safeguards at all stages.

Article 3. Cooperation with other organizations

The two Organizations were to cooperate with other technical assistance and funding agencies concerned, both within and outside the United Nations system, and inform them of this joint approach, with a view to requesting their collaboration in encouraging governments to incorporate health safeguards through the adoption of suitable design and management criteria at the stage of project formulation and approval. The readiness of WHO to advise on such health safeguards was to be brought to the attention of such agencies.

In view of the interest shown by the United Nations Environment Programme in this joint FAO/WHO cooperation, the two Organizations were to inform UNEP of meetings and proposals for action in which UNEP might wish to participate, including direct field cooperation, preparation and publication of technical guidelines and checklists for health safeguards and water development, and the organization of seminars and workshops on health aspects of agricultural water development.

Representatives of FAO and WHO meet annually but, despite good-will, the agreement has not been carried very far in practical terms. Subsequent agreements have furthered technical cooperation, notably through the creation of the Joint WHO/FAO/UNEP Panel of Experts on Environmental Management.

Implementation failures and options for action

It is apparent that agreements among WHO, FAO and the World Bank are not being effectively implemented at the planning level or in the field.

There are alternative approaches that have rarely been exploited. In many developing countries, informal meetings of donor agency staff are held for the purposes of information exchange and coordination to ensure efficient use of resources; they provide an excellent forum for health inputs in water resources projects.

Another option would be for ministries of health to contact the WHO Regional Offices through country representatives to request WHO participation in the development of health sector plans for water resources projects. Such an approach, which is supported by various resolutions of the World Health Assembly, would ensure that better planning procedures were designed and observed and that financial allo-cations for disease control were included. This would be likely to be welcomed by the donor agencies.

Since pre-project support is not usually provided by the donor or loan agency, innovative sources of funding are required. Ministry of health and WHO funds are unlikely to be sufficient to meet the anticipated demand for consultation, data collection, analysis and the preparation of plans. This is an area of opportunity for supporting agencies. In the long term, health sector plans associated with projects would be supported by designated funds in loans.

World Health Assembly resolutions

In 1982 the thirty-fifth World Health Assembly adopted the following resolution (WHA35.17) on the health implications of development schemes:

> . . . Noting that many development projects carry major potential health hazards and dangers for the environment, and that frequently insufficient resources are made available and/or applied in the planning and imple-mentation of development projects to assess these hazards and to pre-vent their occurrence;

Noting further that, on occasions in the past, the health of populations and the environment have deteriorated as a result of development
projects, especially those involving water resources development;

1. PLEDGES WHO's total commitment to work with Member States, national
and international agencies and financial institutions to incorporate
the necessary preventive measures into development projects to
minimize the risks to the health of populations and the environment;

2. URGES Member States, national and international agencies and financial institutions, in the planning and implementation of development
projects, especially those involving water resources development:

(1) to analyse in detail the possible health hazards and environmental
dangers of existing and proposed development projects;

(2) to incorporate into project plans and their implementation adequate measures to prevent, to the greatest extent possible, the
occurrence of health and environmental hazards;

(3) to make adequate provisions for the implementation of the necessary preventive measures in the financing of the relevant development projects;

3. APPEALS to donor countries and relevant financial institutions to assist
developing countries in the implementation of this resolution.

A decade later the health sectors in many Member States still face the
challenge of mobilizing financial and material resources in order to prevent or reduce morbidity and mortality in water development schemes.

The resolution of 1982 was followed in 1986 by resolution WHA
39.22 (Intersectoral Cooperation in National Strategies) and in 1988 by
resolution WHA 41.15 (International Efforts Towards Sustainable Development) re-emphasizing the importance of health in development. More
recently, a broad statement on sustainable development (resolution WHA
42.26) was adopted in 1989 as WHO's contribution to the International
Efforts Towards Sustainable Development:

... Considering that equitable health development is an essential prerequisite for socioeconomic development and that the sustainable and
equitable use of the world's resources will be of paramount importance
for achieving health for all and for the solution of ecological problems;

Concerned that uncontrolled development and the indiscriminate use
of technology have degraded the environment, and that this increasingly
poses threats to the health of the present and future generations and the
sustainability of the development process itself;

3. URGES Member States:

(1) to establish and evaluate policies and strategies for preventing
adverse effects of development on the environment and on health;

(2) to strengthen their national health programmes in this respect,
particularly for:

(a) meeting basic human health needs in the context of development;

(b) providing health care for specific population groups requiring

> attention in the development process—for example, the urban poor;
>
> (c) preventing diseases resulting from uncontrolled development;
>
> (d) assessing and preventing the environmental health risks arising from uncontrolled development and the indiscriminate use of technology;
>
> (3) to strengthen their national health services to enable them to play an active role in the context of sustainable development;
>
> (4) to adopt appropriate legislation regulating anthropogenic influences on ecological systems;
>
> 4. CALLS ON the international community, including development aid agencies and nongovernmental organizations to increase their support for activities to promote a healthy environment and to control adverse effects of development on the environment and on health; . . .

The resolution also requested the Director-General of WHO to give prominence to the interdependence between development, the environment and health in WHO's programmes.

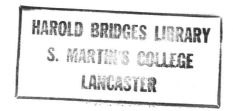

7.

Steps towards solutions

Each developing country has to seek its own ways of providing conditions for satisfactory economic and social development. The steps outlined here lead to policy decisions and derived programmes and action. Policy adjustment is required in order to confront the health hazards associated with development, the direct cost of care and treatment of disease, and the diminishing budgets of health ministries. The steps described address different approaches to achieving policy adjustment.

First principle

The principle has to be established that economic development should not create sickness and disease. Water development projects should allow for health protection at all stages of planning, design, building and operation. This would ensure the evaluation of developmental interventions in their ecological entirety so as to avoid or minimize negative consequences for human health.

Integrated regional planning

Health services should not be developed separately in a water impoundment scheme, but should be an integral part of national and regional health planning and local land-use planning. It is not sufficient to treat disease: health care must be part of a wider development plan for the lake, its surroundings, and broader spheres of influence, the whole being considered as a geographical and economic entity. This approach of integrated regional planning, incorporating health care, also serves the cause of environmental management. Joint consideration should be given to afforestation, the maintenance of fauna and flora, ecosystem stability, the prevention of eutrophication and pollution of lakes and downstream areas by industrial effluents, herbicides and pesticides, and all other environmental effects. Human health cannot be seen as independent of the broader environment.

Incorporation of health costs

Infrastructural costs of health care services and health maintenance should be incorporated into the engineering and public works infrastructural costs of water impoundment schemes. Capital costs thus aggregated reflect total costs in a more realistic way.

After completion of an impoundment scheme, a proportion of its gross income, e.g., 0.5–1% of the gross income from power generation or from cotton or sugar production, should be used to support the costs of health maintenance. Such support should be permanent and should cover the costs of screening, surveillance, prevention, treatment, education, and the control of vectors and intermediate hosts. If this is unacceptable it may be an indication that the economic viability of the project requires re-evaluation.

At one stage the Philippines integrated financial support of disease control measures into new irrigation projects (Tech, 1984). In each of 11 national irrigation projects, covering a total of 265 419 ha, a specific health care budget was indicated for rural health services and the control of malaria and schistosomiasis. Half of the health budgets made up 0.48–5.84% of total project cost in the development period 1983–87, and half covered 13.81–22.30%. Schistosomiasis control has been integrated as a priority programme into the provincial health services, and the National Schistosomiasis Control Service and its infrastructure have been incorporated to provide technical support for the general health services. By 1987 the national prevalence of schistosomiasis was 6.6% and the greatest reductions in prevalence had been achieved in the areas where the International Bank for Reconstruction and Development and the Asian Development Bank had supported schistosomiasis control (Blas, 1989).

Creation of national authorities

New national authorities have been created in the past ten years with responsibility for overseeing water impoundments and irrigation systems, including health promotion. Experiences in Ethiopia, Kenya and the Philippines, and the success achieved by certain binational water development organizations, such as those embracing the frontier river basins of Paraguay and Brazil and of Argentina and Uruguay, suggest that such bodies should have executive power. This requires that they should be created at the highest administrative level, i.e., that of cabinet or presidency, so as to promote cooperation between ministries responsible for public works, power, agriculture, education, health, and transport, and other related bodies. Intersectoral cooperation would be obligatory, subject to the political process. The authority should be constituted so as to work prospectively with more administratively narrow sectoral interests, drawing on the advice of experts in a number of specialist fields—physicians, public health specialists, parasitologists, microbiologists, engineers, biologists, ecologists, agriculturalists, economists and all other sectorally concerned professionals and administrators. It would have the responsibility of setting national goals and priorities for water impoundment and irrigation schemes and would cover both economic interests and health maintenance.

The World Bank now requires that, in all water resources projects financed by the Bank and having major environmental implications, an environmental advisory panel be appointed and that it should meet at least annually. The composition of the panel and its terms of reference are to be described in an environmental reconnaissance report. The panel is expected to function for a few years after the completion of the project. Such a panel may be an important interface with different sectors, including that of health.

Impact assessment

Each proposed scheme should be preceded by a survey, with analysis and evaluation of the findings relating to the potential impact on health as well as to the economic outcome. Such a review would have to be holistic and multidisciplinary. It would identify unintended negative side-effects on health that could be anticipated, and provide cost-benefit analyses of prevention, treatment and control measures. The preparation of appropriate guidelines for such impact assessment should be developed with the collaboration of scientists in developing countries and of international scientific and technical agencies. Since October 1989, such an assessment has been mandatory in all relevant World Bank projects and monitoring is being conducted by the Bank's Department of Environment.

Most major schemes now have environmental assessment integrated into the feasibility stage of planning, and guidelines are available from the World Bank, UNESCO, UNEP and bilateral agencies. The World Bank has a defined policy on dams and reservoirs (Goodland, 1989). In general, the health risks of parasitic diseases are given little attention in these assessments.

Planning for the project area and beyond

Protection of the environment so that water quality is maintained and most of the health risks produced by a water development project are avoided requires appropriate use of the land that is geographically and economically influenced by the project. This means that the use of the land around the impoundment, and the establishment of new settlements and industrial, agricultural or other activities, should be planned and regulated in accordance with ecological principles and sanitary and social interests. This type of planning activity is the most economic and efficient way to prevent or control risks to health, as well as to improve the quality of life in the area. One of the purposes of planning activities is to ensure that a reasonable part of the investment and of the benefits produced by a water resources project goes to finance and guide local development.

Monitoring, evaluation and response

An essential part of policy implementation is to generate a capacity to respond to problems as they arise. A continuing programme that monitors ecosystem and health data with specific lines of reporting and administrative mechanisms for action should be incorporated into each water resources project. The monitoring may cover flora, fauna, hydrology, agriculture, and human social and health conditions. The investigations would be on a small scale and modestly funded. Continuing evaluations of control efforts associated with large and small impoundments should be integrated with planning strategies in a research feedback loop.

In large institutionalized schemes a multidisciplinary unit could be established to investigate and improve disease control. Except during the special circumstances of an epidemic, health protection requires the presence of a multidisciplinary team that has a defined programme of work and a schedule of activities. Moreover, it should have the administrative authority to initiate surveys, interpret data, and plan and coordinate programmes for the prevention or control of disease risks.

Above all it should have responsibility for making recommendations on environment and health to the administration of the scheme. Such a team, using suitable ecological and epidemiological techniques, should be able to estimate disease risks with sufficient precision to recommend, if necessary, essential changes in the plans of the water resources project or in the organization and use of land so as to eliminate or minimize the dangers. The team should be represented in every major water resources project or group of projects under the same authority from the very beginning. It should be permanent and represented at the decision-making level.

In most countries it would be feasible for qualified persons in the ministry of health or the national agency coordinating water resources development to manage these activities in collaboration with national research institutions.

Integrated development strategies

Multisectoral planning

Only through integrated, multisectoral planning, evolving around the water impoundment scheme, is it possible to achieve the goals of power production, increased agricultural production and improved health.

Guidelines

Guidelines on integrated development planning, eventually leading to specific technical manuals, should cover health planning. Health guidelines should be concise, explicit and widely applicable, and should include recommendations for the creation of multidisciplinary planning teams. Technical manuals that are developed subsequently should be multidisciplinary and strongly integrated by the application of systems methodology.

Intersectoral coordination

It is necessary to integrate sectoral planning for agronomics, ecology, economics, environmental monitoring, epidemiology, health services, clinics, health surveillance, housing, hygiene, hydrology, limnology, social activity, vector biology, wildlife ecology, and unplanned or 'spontaneous' settlements.

Regional coordination

Just as intersectoral coordination is required in integrated development planning, regional or spatial coordination is equally necessary. In the spatial sense an integration of planning should be effected between areas above and below the dam, around the impoundment in the different parts of the watershed, and beyond watershed boundaries. Impoundment projects typically affect the migration of populations from distant areas, new marketing zones, and the national economy.

Cost synthesis

Along with regional and sectoral coordination, cost synthesis should be effected by aggregating all components of infrastructural costs with the components of operational and maintenance costs. Appropriate health-related costs for such aggregation should be identified in all the different sectors of the scheme, such as water impoundment, agricultural production, housing and population activity, and vector biology and control.

National standards

National regulations

An environmental impact statement, including reference to effects on social matters and health is now considered a prerequisite by most international financial or development agencies for the authorization and continuation of planning. The proposed strategies for integrated development should conform to national guidelines or regulations where these exist.

Countries should develop regulations to cover the continuous evaluation of the health impact and other effects of impoundment schemes after their construction. In other words the regulations should extend beyond the initial creation of schemes to their long-term operation.

National registration

There is a growing awareness of the need to understand both current and projected growth rates in the construction of large and small water impoundment schemes. A lack of information on these developments becomes increasingly disquieting to health officials confronted by the disease effects of water impoundments. Data are lacking on numbers, size and other specific characteristics of impoundments and irrigation schemes, including engineering, hydrological, agricultural and human health characteristics. Specific quantitative data should be collected on a continuing basis.

Water-related ecological phenomena linked to human diseases, zoonoses and vectors need to be identified. A national register would assist in this respect and in the recognition of specific problems. A functional topology categorizing impoundments with different purposes would help to identify problems, priorities and needs in the promotion of health services and disease research. International assistance and coordination are needed in the development of national registers.

Use of remote sensing and geographical information systems

In most developing countries no single ministry or agency has a registry of the total number and geographical locations of man-made bodies of water, or even of those constructed by the authorities. This is a serious impediment to risk assessment for health services planning.

Aerial photography at a suitable scale can be useful in the preparation of a geographical listing of dams, but coverage is incomplete, the available pictures are usually out of date, and the technique is expensive. Alternatively, remote satellite sensing, with improved-resolution imagery, holds the greatest promise of affordable, rapidly renewable coverage. At the simplest level it can indicate the numbers and locations of impoundments and can facilitate the calculation of their surface areas. The method is efficient, inexpensive and comprehensive. It could also be used, for example, in the design of field investigations of disease.

Since satellite coverage serves all sectors of the national economy, its cost would not be a responsibility of ministries of health alone. Technical planning information is available from the UNEP Global Resources Information Database.[a] FAO's Land and Water Resources Division also has technical expertise in this area.

Techniques for the analysis of large numbers of observations, all spatially characterized, are now available for use in personal computers. This type of analysis is essential in exploiting the data collected by the above techniques as well as the health and environmental data collected in the field. A wide range of new geographical information systems software is particularly suitable for health management problems and for multisectoral integrative analysis. In practice the application of these techniques to health has been largely unexplored.

---

[a] Global Resources Information Database, 6 rue de la Gabelle, 1227 Carouge, Switzerland.

Financial support

Conditional financing

Applications for international grants and loans for water development projects should be carefully scrutinized by national and donor agencies to ensure that they conform to national regulations for health promotion. The drawing up of plans for integrated development may constitute a prior condition for applications for loans from the World Bank and other international financing bodies in the future. The disbursement of nationally generated funds for impoundment schemes should also comply with the desired conditions; this is already becoming standard practice.

Debt for health

The massive debt of developing countries has placed an even greater onus on the productivity and economic return of current investment. The "debt for nature" exchanges will produce modest national conservation budgets, depending on the extent to which forest owners' debts are discounted on the secondary debt market (Goodland et al., 1990). These exchanges do not mean *a priori* that inflation will ensue, but sovereignty is maintained. Likewise a "debt for health" exchange could be envisaged. The declining budgets of ministries of health are widely recognized (WHO Regional Office for South-East Asia, 1989). The surveillance and maintenance of control of parasitic diseases require extensive long-term resources. This option needs to be explored and encouraged by that part of the international financial community concerned with development.

Infrastructural costs of health care

Capital costs of the necessary health care infrastructure, such as for buildings, clinics, outpatient facilities and so on, should be included in the integrated capital costs of projects. In addition, the costs of recruiting and training teams of health care professionals for rural areas should be included at the outset. In developing countries, additional health care personnel are not, as a rule, immediately available to meet the extra demands created by new projects, and a training scheme is normally needed.

Recurring costs for health services, screening, treatment, vector control and health education should be covered in standard budget planning. The funds required for recurrent operational expenditure should be derived directly or indirectly from gross income. This should be done as needed or on some equivalency basis, for instance by taking a fixed proportion of project income. Recurrent costs should also include those of regular health surveillance and evaluation and of environmental monitoring.

In macroeconomic terms, developing countries that use their own resources to control parasitic diseases may not require structural adjustment. On the other hand, if the control of parasitic diseases is dependent on government subsidies, as, for example, with subsidized pesticides, structural adjustment lending may introduce reforms to reduce them (World Bank/International Monetary Fund, 1989). Subsidies of this type may represent misallocations of health resources, and should not be considered in the same way as subsidies in other sectors. The strategy and the size of the target areas should be commensurate with the national capacity to finance the control activities. A hidden pitfall of low-cost additional financing is its negative effect on the development of self-reliance and long-term sustainability. Unfortunately, the desire for rapid achievement may overwhelm the rationale of a long-term strategy that does not offer spectacular results.

Innovative national financing options should be considered, among them differential taxation schemes, tax rebates or reductions, and employer insurance schemes. Their feasibility depends on the economic and political frameworks of the countries concerned.

8.
Intersectoral negotiating strategies for health authorities

Each country and each water development project is unique in its disease profile, environmental context, biological diversity and social and economic setting. The countries of South-East Asia, West Africa, the Eastern Mediterranean and South America differ from one other, and their national needs, resources and planning responses vary accordingly. The present chapter cannot cover every need and contingency, but it can be used selectively according to particular requirements. It offers a framework in which options can be evaluated as a basis for well-informed decision-making. This is a corollary of the recommendation of the Bangalore Symposium (WHO Regional Office for South-East Asia, 1989) that the capacities of ministries of health should be strengthened so that development projects can be analysed to ensure that they do not have a negative impact on health status. This chapter is intended to provide a strategy framework for ministries of health to ensure the correct identification of problems and the submission of feasible proposals for prevention and control to the sectors responsible for project approval and implementation. This information needs to be communicated to policy-makers so that policy adjustments can be made. At the political level, legal frameworks should be developed to safeguard health status in water resources projects.

The constraints affecting ministries of health within government administrations are implicit throughout. Health is one of the most politically visible and sensitive of all public issues. Water resources projects attract close scrutiny; they are viewed by governments as the key to economic development, by environmentalists as a potential ecological threat, and by health authorities with caution. Whenever an epidemic or other health crisis is announced, the ministry of health has to respond. If the budget and manpower for surveillance and monitoring have been inadequate for a long time the response is likely to be delayed, uncoordinated and palliative. Such a short-term and short-sighted approach cannot build a base for future monitoring or a permanent capability for action.

Awareness of disease effects and economic loss

Economists, engineers, agronomists and other technical and financial planning professionals usually have an inadequate understanding of the costs of diseases, and of the benefits of prevention, and often lack first-hand experience of the suffering and incapacity produced by water-related diseases. As a result the costs of ill health tend to be ignored. However, if such people were given the opportunity to observe the effects of clinical disease, due weight might be accorded to preventive measures in development planning. Common ground should be established in intersectoral presentations and discussions. Illustrative materials can be supplied by WHO to help communication with target groups. These could include information on clinical matters, physical incapacity, loss of days at school and work, reduced agricultural production, chronic morbidity, and death. However, data from national sources are often the most convincing in the intersectoral dialogue. In this respect, national medical research institutions can be supported by government and other agencies.in research that is in harmony with development needs.

Beyond culpability

Health officials need to be actively involved in the planning and implementation of water resources projects. The first step is to go to the other sectors. The second is to show, either outside or within water resources projects, that the prevention and control of parasitic diseases are feasible. The traditional passive position of the health sector is so widely expected that proposals may initially be treated sceptically. In order to make progress there should be no attempt to apportion blame for omitting the health sector from past discussions.

Obtaining information on new and proposed water development schemes

Intersectoral dialogue cannot proceed with equity if ministries of health receive information only after projects have been established (WHO, 1986a). Large numbers of village dams may be built without local or national health authorities being given any advance notice of their location. Even in major projects, technical information essential for health planning is not usually disseminated, even though it is available at the feasibility stage. Links with coordinating agencies at this stage can assist in obtaining the information required.

Forewarned health authorities can be forearmed to become proactive rather than reactive. The health sector is likely to be poorly represented in intersectoral policy discussions and in implementation if it receives information on water resources development only after construction has taken place. Thus ministries of health should create their own information systems on water schemes, develop liaison and personal lines of communication with the executing agencies, assign personnel, and create routine procedures to secure advance knowledge of the nature, scale, location and range of activities in development projects. Administrative agreements on linkages between sectors of government should be established.

The project cycle

Donor and lending organizations are led by the World Bank, regional development banks, UNDP, donor countries, and bilateral assistance programmes. The diversity of these organizations is such that there is no single type of project cycle. One example is that of the World Bank (Baum, 1982), in which the process of bringing a development project to fruition involves the following steps.

- **Identification**
  National and sectoral potential; credit-worthiness; prima facie feasibility; environmental reconnaissance study; costs commensurate with expected benefits. This stage may take several months.
- **Preparation**
  Prepared by the borrower: project brief; objectives; issues; timetable; technical, institutional, economic and financial analysis; resources investigation; technical package; government policies; alternatives. The engineering feasibility study is completed. This stage usually evolves over two to three years.
- **Appraisal**
  Comprehensive review of all aspects; lays foundations for implementation and evaluation. Momentum builds up and this stage may take only two months.
  — *Technical*: design; scale; layout; location of facilities; equipment; cost estimates; physical contingencies. The potential impact of the project on the human and physical environment is examined to make sure that any adverse effects will be controlled or minimized.

111

— *Institutional*: institution building; management capability and initiative; policies and procedures.
— *Economic*: cost-benefit analysis of alternative designs; sectoral setting; strengths and weaknesses of sectoral institutions; economic rate of return; "shadow" prices; distribution of benefits; "social" prices.
— *Financial*: sufficiency of funds; co-financing; development banks; bilateral aid agencies; rates of return; financial viability; debt-to-equity ratios; price-revenue policies; recovery of investment and operating costs; interest rates.

- **Negotiations, board presentation**
  Agreements; terms of loan; legal obligations; financial covenant; project unit administration. This stage takes a minimum of two months.
- **Implementation and supervision**
  Construction; operation; implementation pathway variations; design and operations feedback; monitoring and review; progress reports; procurement of goods and works; consultant services. On average this stage lasts five years.
- **Evaluation**
  (*Ex-post facto* audit; impact evaluation report; lessons for identification, design and preparation of future projects. It takes eight to ten years to complete the cycle.

Environmental assessment in the project cycle

All donor agencies are now developing, if not implementing, policies on environment and health, ranging from health impact assessment to prevention and mitigation.

In 1989 the World Bank promulgated a new official policy on projects related to dams and reservoirs for hydropower generation, irrigation or water supply. Procedures are designed to ensure that environmental requirements become integrated into project design and operation. The overall aim is to promote projects with the lowest possible environmental and social costs (Goodland, 1989). During project identification, an environmental reconnaissance is performed by independent recognized experts or firms selected by the borrower and approved by the Bank. This aims to identify potential environmental effects, to ascertain the scope of further environmental studies and actions needed, to assess the ability of the borrower to undertake these studies and to advise on the need for an environmental panel (World Bank, 1989).

The World Bank has also adopted a policy on environmental assessment which includes consideration of the impacts of projects on health (World Bank/International Monetary Fund, 1987, 1988, 1989). Such recognition of the linkages between health, environment and development has not generally been emphasized by borrowing countries or supported by specific health action plans for "preventive, mitigatory and compensatory measures" (World Bank, 1989).

Health sector involvement in the cycle

Full participation of the health sector in all stages of the cycle, including pre-cycle explorations, is necessary if public health in the vicinity of proposed impoundments is to be safeguarded. Qualified staff located in ministries of health should be designated to represent the public health viewpoint. These persons should fully understand the project cycle schemas of international financing agencies, and, when appropriate, of the regional banks and bilateral assistance programmes. Direct involvement at all phases of technical and financial planning is advantageous. The expression of health sector concerns, introduced with technical and organizational options, forms part of the process of negotiation.

Project health care is most appropriately managed by ministries of health with a permanent presence on site. For large projects the World Bank requires an on-site environmental unit. The corresponding unit for health can be proposed in the health sector plan by the ministry of health. The ministry or agency executing the project then ensures that financial support is included in the budget proposal.

Financial support for health protection

The objective of health sector participation in intersectoral negotiation is to secure funds within the water development project for health maintenance activities. In the preparation phase these cover consultants, surveys and training. Start up, infrastructure and recurring operational costs should be included in the project loan. In past water development schemes effective health care management has been absent because of a lack of comprehensive planning by the health sector. Rarely has the financial commitment been refused if a plan has been presented. Alternative sources of funding include grants or revenues issued directly to the health unit within the project, or indirectly via the ministry of health.

Improved intersectoral cooperation

The provision of funds for health care establishes a new basis for intersectoral collaboration in health promotion. One can envisage that a ministry of education would emphasize health education measures in school curricula, to try to change health-related behaviour; that a ministry of social work would initiate non-formal health education for adults and engage in community health programmes; and that a ministry of agriculture would become involved in cleaning channels and other measures for vector control. An intersectoral coordinating agency could be established to fund these health activities with resources derived from lending agencies and government, and directed solely to the mitigation of ecological and health problems.

Nongovernmental organizations

Private and nongovernmental groups, such as churches and missions, play an important role in health education and the provision of medical services in numerous developing countries. Many of these groups also promote water resources development without consultation with government. In some areas they may usefully contribute to intersectoral discussions on the planning, design and implementation of water projects. The support of nongovernmental organizations as forceful advocates for health promotion and protection in water resources projects can be coordinated by the ministry of health.

The basis of the negotiating strategy in water resources projects

Summary of arguments

The principle arguments for the involvement of the ministry of health in intersectoral negotiations are as follows.

- An understanding of the ecology and epidemiology of water-related diseases permits a clearer choice of options for project implementation.
- Specification of the disease risk to which the productive labour force is exposed creates an awareness of the need for preventive measures.

- There is a close relationship between good water management practices and both economic and health outcomes.
- High-quality health services in project areas can have a beneficial effect on the health of populations in surrounding areas.
- Effective health surveillance and monitoring systems, allowing early detection of schistosomiasis transmission and recognition of malaria or hepatitis epidemics, help maintain the capacity of the work force.
- Existing technologies can be harnessed for control strategies that are both feasible and effective.

Presentation of arguments

Each argument should be explored in detail by health ministry representatives with a view to articulating it in language that can be understood by all the professionals involved.

Argument 1. An understanding of the ecology and epidemiology of water-related diseases permits a clearer choice of options for project implementation

Health ministries have the most accurate information on the distribution of waterborne diseases. Areas of similar ecology do not necessarily have the same disease endemicity. It may be useful to propose project implementation in nonendemic rather than in highly endemic areas with attendant risks.

Furthermore, disease distributions among migrant populations likely to be involved in projects, from the construction phase to the operational phase, should be ascertained.

If such data are not available, health ministries may propose specific interventions to be carried out at the same time as the data are being collected. This is particularly true in the case of schistosomiasis, for which safe effective oral treatment can be given at the time of diagnosis. Urinary schistosomiasis can be diagnosed using simple chemical reagent strips to detect haematuria, or by simple questionnaire. Malaria and filariasis control can be initiated by specific interventions against the vectors. Treatment is also available for acute malaria, whereby morbidity and mortality can be immediately reduced in the project area.

Argument 2. Potential disease risk and need for prevention

Preventive measures should be paramount. If preventive measures are taken sufficiently early, they require fewer personnel, less equipment, and

115

less material than do curative measures taken after the breeding areas of disease vectors or intermediate hosts have expanded and the prevalence rates of diseases have increased.

Available estimates can be used to forecast the effects of diseases on the workers and the people involved in all phases of the project and in all areas affected.

Schistosomiasis

Infection (no evidence of severe disease). 26–42 working days lost per year in the Philippines due to *S. japonicum* (Blas, 1989); 4.4 working days lost per year due to *S. haematobium* (Ghana Health Assessment Team, 1981; Morrow, 1984). In Madagascar, 50% of people reported as unable to work had evidence of urinary schistosomiasis, and remained out of work for 10 days (Breuil et al., 1983a); 6 working days are lost per year due to *S. mansoni* infection (Chowdhury & Levy, 1988). Absenteeism among sugarcane workers infected with *S. mansoni* was found to be twice as high as among uninfected workers (Ndamba et al., 1991). Single-dose treatment of an adult costs less than US$ 1.

Disease. There is a latent period of 5–15 years between infection and severe disease. Hepatosplenomegaly due to *S. mansoni* occurs in persons aged over 20 years. Approximately 10% of those infected develop irreversible pathological changes of the liver.

An 18% reduction in the work output of persons with severe disease can be expected (Awad El Karim et al., 1980); those with infection only may have no reduction of work output (van Ee & Polderman, 1984). Of those with hepatosplenomegaly, 33% have oesophageal varices (De Cock et al., 1982). Once oesophageal varices have started to bleed, this tends to recur, leading to the loss of 3–4 months a year, either in or out of hospital.

Disease of the central nervous system, affecting the spinal cord, is more frequent and causes more disability than currently appreciated, especially among migrants who enter areas where *S. mansoni* is endemic (WHO, 1989b; Joubert et al., 1990).

A reduction in exercise capacity of at least 12% was found in children with *S. haematobium* infection in Zimbabwe (Ndamba, 1986); recovery occurred one month after treatment. Similarly, a 7–10% improvement in exercise capacity was found in children with *S. haematobium* infection one month after treatment in Kenya (Latham et al., 1990).

If a person with schistosomiasis acquires intercurrent typhoid fever, the duration of the latter is 2–3 times the average; the disease may lead to total incapacity and death in up to 30% of untreated persons (WHO, 1989b).

The duration of intercurrent hepatitis B is up to five times the average; there is an increased risk of chronic liver disease and sequelae, and total incapacity may occur (Ghaffar et al., 1990). Furthermore there is a decreased response to hepatitis B vaccine (Bassily et al., 1987; Ghaffar et al., 1990).

Malaria

In acute malaria each episode of *Plasmodium falciparum* infection costs at least seven days of work lost (Ghana Health Assessment Team, 1981). With appropriate treatment this may be reduced to four or five days. The cost of a single treatment of nonresistant malaria is US$ 0.10; the treatment of resistant malaria may cost up to US$ 60 for the drugs alone.

In recurrent malaria the frequency of recurrence depends on the effectiveness of the original treatment, the risk of reinfection as measured by mosquito density and exposure, and the immune status of the individual. The risk of infection can be reduced by personal measures of protection: mosquito nets costing up to US$ 2 a year and chemoprophylaxis costing US$ 1 per person per year.

Filariasis

Acute infection is associated with fever, urticaria and recurrent lymphangitis. Each infected adult male can be expected to lose 3–15 days of work a year due to scrotal, inguinal or axillary lymphangitis. These episodes may occur two or three times a year. Treatment costs up to $ 0.25.

In cases of chronic infection, elephantiasis of the scrotum, leg or arm develops within 1–2 years after infection in immigrants from non-endemic areas. This leads to total incapacity and exclusion from the work force. Rates of chronic infection are directly proportional to the prevalence of infection (WHO, 1992a).

Onchocerciasis

The annual incidence of blindness due to onchocerciasis is 4–7 per 1000 infected persons. The peak onset is at 39 years of age and life expectancy is less than 49 years. The prevalence of blindness is up to 15% in savanna localities and up to 2% in forest villages. Treatment with ivermectin costs US$ 3.

Argument 3. Close relationship between good water management practices and both economic and health outcomes

Good water management practices can be justified on economic, agronomic and energy conservation grounds (Schramm & Warford, 1989).

Ministries of health need to understand and recognize that professional engineering competence in the design and maintenance of irrigation systems, small reservoirs and large dams will assist in the control of waterborne diseases. In this crucial intersectoral aspect of water resources development, health ministries can provide support and justification to ministries of agriculture or energy for adequate design and management, if unacceptable short-cuts are proposed at the higher planning levels. Specific designs and maintenance procedures have been evaluated under field conditions for their ability to contribute to reducing the numbers of vectors of waterborne diseases. Sadly, recommendations developed in this specialized area have not been widely recognized or implemented by the international civil engineering community. Poor water management and inadequate maintenance of irrigation systems are the bane of the irrigated agricultural sector (see McJunkin, 1975; Pike, 1987; Oomen et al., 1988, 1990).

Argument 4. The beneficial effect of high-quality health services on the health of populations in surrounding areas

The physical infrastructure of health care facilities in a project may present an opportunity to extend comprehensive health services to neighbouring populations in an entire district or subregion. Financial resources for the project can support the creation of an infrastructure for a major part of the surrounding district and best use can be made of government resources in employing and training staff and in building the physical infrastructure outside the project area.

Argument 5. Effective health surveillance and monitoring systems help maintain the capacity of the work force

The current epidemiological surveillance capacities of health ministries in developing countries are, almost without exception, uneven and slow to react to change or to epidemics. Such surveillance is one of the key public health activities of a health authority, yet it often has a low priority in health ministries.

Communication aimed at forcing action against an epidemic usually takes place through the media or political circles. Water resources projects create epidemiological conditions conducive to epidemics of acute diseases or to rapid increases in the prevalence of chronic parasitic infections. If the advance warning systems of projects are used to monitor data from inpatient and outpatient health services, as well as data on vector populations, they can help to avoid the introduction, spread and aggravation of parasitic diseases. Such systems can be polyvalent and need not be confined to the untoward effects of parasitic diseases.

In terms of surveillance, project areas should not be considered in geographical isolation. Diseases introduced into project areas may be traceable to surrounding areas, sometimes at great distances, where intervention may be necessary to avoid further spread. Moreover, project areas may be important foci for the dissemination of diseases and vectors. An efficient surveillance system in a water resources project has both short- and long-term economic benefits in reducing morbidity and mortality, and a project can often serve as a regional or national model for achieving this goal.

Argument 6. Existing technologies can be harnessed for feasible and effective control strategies

The control of parasitic diseases today aims first and foremost to reduce morbidity and mortality, and the tools needed for this purpose are available.

Operationally, malaria control requires correct diagnosis of fever caused by the disease, adequate treatment of the acute condition, vector control according to the ecological setting, environmental management, and personal protection (e.g., with bednets).

For schistosomiasis the control strategy is based on diagnosis of infection, treatment focused on children of school age and workers, selective snail control in places where people become infected, provision of community water supplies, and avoidance of contact with natural bodies of water for domestic and recreational activities.

Filariasis control is focused on early diagnosis and the treatment of infection to avoid severe disease, together with adequate mosquito control.

Onchocerciasis control is aimed at detecting and eliminating the breeding sites of *Simulium* (blackflies), either by environmental modification or by the use of insecticides. This can be combined with mass treatment with ivermectin to reduce the numbers of microfilariae in the blood and to reduce transmission.

It is noteworthy that once the severe form of any of the above diseases develops in an individual, treatment becomes extremely difficult. The management of severe malaria, for example, requires advanced clinical skills and an adequate hospital infrastructure.

All of these diseases are controllable. Of course, improvements can be expected in the future, but the existing means of treatment and control are technically feasible and economically affordable in relation to the potential economic benefits of projects.

9.

How to develop a health plan for a water resources project

Primary planning goals

Given the growth of water resources development for the purposes of agriculture and energy production, clear planning goals should be adopted in order to mitigate adverse health consequences. The keys to success are a well-prepared, operationally feasible and affordable plan, and sustained financial support. In particular, the project health plan should:

— ensure that analysis of the impact on health becomes an essential part of project appraisal;
— incorporate the cost of disease control into the project's budget;
— develop appropriate methods for surveillance and monitoring of health status, including early warning of emerging health hazards, and ensure that they are employed during the implementation of the project;
— train local health workers to identify and treat emerging health problems;
— make people aware of problems using existing systems of information, education and communication;
— maintain health profiles of both local and migrant populations in the project area so that appropriate health interventions can be devised;
— promote the formation of local, private, nongovernmental and voluntary organizations, including traditional village groups, to assist in implementing the project health plan.

Practical steps

In formulating the project health plan, officials of the ministry of health should:

— review the existing health care infrastructure, and the staff and resources available;

— identify endemic diseases and vectors;
— make a risk assessment and a projection of health hazards;
— make a list of medical needs for the treatment of schistosomiasis, malaria and filariasis, with reference to infrastructure, supplies and the timing and phasing of the programme;
— identify personnel needs and devise recruitment and training programmes;
— estimate the financial costs of the above activities for start-up survey and training activities, and for continuation of the programme.

Technical components for the project health plan and its implementation are suggested in the Annex.

Budget planning should be fully developed to include cost-sharing arrangements, if any, with other government ministries and agencies, amortization, contingencies and, especially, long-term financial support. The budget should reflect the operational plan and should be realistically constructed in relation to the resources available and to competing needs.

If a budget for health is included in the project, its use by the ministry of health will be optimized by efficient management and appropriate forward planning. It is recognized that health ministries in developing countries are often subject to crisis management and action in support of political objectives. However, by being given financial support and direct executive responsibility for public health interventions in water resources projects, the ministries have an opportunity to show that their role is merited and to create confidence for future projects.

Pre-project health risk assessment

In the earliest phase of planning, the ministry of health should provide an analysis of the prevailing distributions and epidemiological significance of parasitic diseases in the proposed development area. Existing surveillance data may be used, or rapid evaluation surveys of risk undertaken, using either the ministry's own staff and resources or national institutions contracted for the purpose. Foreign consultants may be invited to prepare an assessment, but this is usually the least satisfactory solution because of a lack of long-term contact with the country and the people, and because secondary documents and reports may be interpreted without orientation to the project site.

Health impact assessments are becoming routine for the approval of water resources projects by funding agencies. However, even when required as part of the project document, such assessments are usually descriptive rather than prescriptive; if prescriptive, their medical orientation is clinical rather than preventive. A well prepared risk assessment study is indispensable for estimating sustainability, modifying the project design, and anticipating needs for health services.

Project cycle information on health risk assessment, data management, budget planning and operational methods is being generated continuously by donor and lending agencies; this information, collated and synthesized in a variety of short formats, would be very useful to health authorities in developing countries. Accessible databases on low-cost personal computer diskettes would greatly assist health ministry officials in risk assessment, project planning, and programme monitoring and management. In-country, in-service workshops would facilitate the transfer of this technology.

Integrated control

The project health plan may consider: integration of control into the primary health care system; integration with control of other diseases; and intersectoral collaboration aimed at identifying how other sectors can contribute to disease control. Such integration would improve cost-effectiveness, and make the most of the resources available to the ministry of health. Intersectoral cooperation for improved disease control is an essential planning goal rather than an option. The main areas of cooperation would be in sanitation, water supply and agriculture.

A recent meeting (WHO, 1989a) on strategies to reduce morbidity caused by schistosomiasis recognized both the difficulties and the potential of integrated control, and concluded that control would be best maintained through the general health care services. It recommended that diagnosis, treatment, and epidemiological reporting should be available at the village level. Experiences in Botswana, Guinea, Pemba, and the Philippines have illustrated different aspects of the problem of involvement of health services ranging from lack of trained staff, inadequate infrastructure without supervision, inappropriate job descriptions and absence of operational guidelines. In spite of the lack of well-documented successes, these efforts must continue so as to provide experience necessary for future programmes.

There is a consensus that integration with control of other diseases may be a necessity in the face of diminishing resources of ministries of health, but experience is limited. In Morocco, the integrated community surveys of schistosomiasis and malaria have been operational for more than ten years, primarily in irrigated areas. Intestinal parasite control is a feasible integration option and is appreciated at the community level. However, the priorities at higher administrative levels, and in the donor agencies, rarely include intestinal parasites. More experience is required to determine the feasibility of the integration of schistosomiasis control with that of malaria, leishmaniasis, filariasis and dracunculiasis.

There is also a consensus that the impact of chemotherapy can be optimized by the presence of a water supply. Cure rates are higher and intervals between retreatments are longer when an adequate safe water supply is present.

WHO's Community Water Supply and Sanitation Unit, evaluating data on the status of the Water Decade, emphasized the preventive potential of water supply programmes especially regarding schistosomiasis (WHO, 1989a). Water supply programmes may be used to orientate implementation in areas where the effect on schistosomiasis can be demonstrated. Health staff should be encouraged to pursue this matter at the outset of water supply projects and to back up implementation with increased health education efforts. The health concepts should relate to diseases associated with water supply. While maintenance of water supplies is generally problematic, it is felt that the monitoring of usage as well as of health indicators, together with health education, may effectively promote maintenance.

Progressively polyvalent control strategies

Efforts should be made to control a number of diseases, such as schistosomiasis, malaria, leishmaniasis, filariasis and dracunculiasis, at the same time in the same programme. An allocation of scarce resources to control a single disease is short-sighted if measures against other diseases can be included.

Either initially multiple or progressively multiple control activities may be appropriate for different development projects. An initially multiple approach may be applicable where one disease is predominant and others are not of significant public health importance. More frequently, several diseases are important according to various criteria but human and financial resources are not sufficient to combat all of them simultaneously. In such circumstances, a priority ranking and a sequence of activities should be developed.

Priority ranking can be achieved by asking the following questions. Is the technology for control available? Is the technology simple, and can health personnel be easily trained in its application? Is the technology amenable to quality control and evaluation? What is the time interval between application of the technology and the earliest possible detection of its impact? Does the disease affect or threaten the majority of the population in the project area?

The multiple-disease approach has been appropriate in the Gezira, Sudan, and in Beni Mellal Province, Morocco, where both malaria and schistosomiasis are public health problems. On the island of Pemba, United Republic of Tanzania, although malaria is the major problem, resources are limited and schistosomiasis has been selected as the initial target, with time-limited objectives for progressive inclusion of control measures against intestinal parasites, malaria and filariasis. The fact that 20% of the island's surface is water qualifies it for consideration as a large-scale water resources project.

Conclusions

The catalogue of adverse health effects of parasitic diseases in water resources development continues to grow. The list of new and proposed projects in which there are predictably high risks of malaria, schistoso-miasis, filariasis and onchocerciasis is longer and more diverse than ever before. The basic tenets of the economic development process are being questioned and critically scrutinized by the international financing community and by the countries involved. There is a widespread awareness of the dangers of environmental degradation, but it is not certain that the associated health issues will be adequately tackled. The present difficulties of health ministries are interrelated and hinder health programmes in water resources projects.

This book is a call for health ministries to enter the project cycle of water resources development. Their potential role can no longer be ignored. Development cannot be expected automatically to confine its harmful impact on health to socially, economically or even politically acceptable levels. The negotiating strategies presented here should help ministries of health to enter effectively into the project cycle.

Ministries of health should prepare operational plans for the utilization of external resources available to projects, in order to improve general health services and to achieve disease prevention and control. The re-sponsibilities of all parties concerned should be agreed so as to ensure coordinated implementation. If a physical infrastructure is to be built, then supplies, equipment and staff must be planned, and administrative procedures initiated, before construction begins. The time required for the procurement of supplies and equipment and for the selection, employ-ment, training and placement of staff equals that needed for the construc-tion of the physical infrastructure. Preparations for the supervision and monitoring of health activities should begin at the outset of the planning process. This vital function of health ministries is usually weak or absent in health care delivery systems of developing countries. The health care system of a water resources project can be the opportunity to create effective planning mechanisms and an epidemiological surveillance network for the first time. This step cannot be taken as an afterthought, since it is one of the key components of the negotiating strategy.

The potential for water resources development impinges on all areas of economic development. Parasitic diseases are one aspect of health within the development process. The available tools and our understanding of the epidemiology, prevention and control of these diseases, although not complete, are sufficient to justify action.

References

Abdallah A, ed. (1978) *Proceedings of the International Conference on Schistosomiasis, Cairo, 1975.* Cairo, Ministry of Health.

Abdel-Wahab MF et al. (1979) Changing patterns of schistosomiasis in Egypt, 1935–1979. *Lancet,* **2**: 242–244.

Abisudjak B, Kotanegara R (1989) Transmigration and vector-borne diseases in Indonesia. In: Service MW, ed., *Demography and vector-borne diseases,* Boca Raton, FL, CRC Press, pp. 207–223.

Ackermann WC, White GF, Worthington EB (1973) *Man-made lakes: their problems and environmental effects.* Washington, DC, American Geophysical Union (Geophysical Monograph Series No. 17).

Ackers GL, Smith DH (1988) Design and management of development projects to avoid health hazards. *Journal of tropical medicine and hygiene,* **91**: 115–129.

Adekolu-John EO (1979a) A communication on health and development in the Kainji Lake area of Nigeria. *Acta tropica,* **36**: 91–102.

Adekolu-John EO (1979b) The role of dispensaries in community health care in the Kainji Lake area of Nigeria. *Journal of epidemiology and community health,* **33**: 145–149.

Adekolu-John EO (1980) The probable impact of the proposed Jebba Dam on the health aspects of the River Niger Basin of Nigeria. *Public health,* **94**: 235–242.

Adekolu-John EO (1983) *A health survey of the people of Kainji Lake area of Nigeria.* Ibadan, Nigeria, University of Ibadan (MD Thesis).

Adekolu-John EO, Abolarin O (1986) Status of human schistosomiasis on the eastern side of Kainji Lake area of Nigeria. *East African medical journal,* **63** (7): 463–470.

Adekolu-John EO, Fagbami AH (1983) Arthropod-borne virus antibodies in sera of residents of Kainji Lake Basin, Nigeria, 1980. *Transactions of the Royal Society of Tropical Medicine and Hygiene,* **77** (2): 149–151.

Agadzi VK (1986) *Trypanosomiasis in Ghana.* Geneva, World Health Organization (unpublished document).

Alexandratos N (1988) *World agriculture: toward 2000. An FAO study.* London, Belhaven Press/Pinter Publishers.

Alexis L (1986) Sri Lanka's Mahaweli Ganga Project: the damnation of paradise. In: Goldsmith E, Hildyard N, eds, *The social and environmental effects of large dams. Vol. 2. Case studies.* Camelford, Cornwall, Wadebridge Ecological Centre.

Amin MA (1977) Problems and effects of schistosomiasis in irrigation schemes in the Sudan. In: Worthington EB, ed., *Arid land irrigation in developing countries. Environmental problems and effects.* Oxford, Pergamon Press, pp. 407–411.

Andrade RM de (1969) Nota ecologica sobre o Lago de Pampulha (Belo Horizonte MG), com especial refêrencia aos planorbideos (Pulmonata, Planorbidae). *Revista brasileira de malariologia e doenças tropicais*, **21**: 59–116.

Arfaa F et al. (1970) Progress towards the control of bilharziasis in Iran. *Transactions of the Royal Society of Tropical Medicine and Hygiene*, **64**: 912–917.

Arfaa F (1988a) *Schistosomiasis prevention and control in Jordan*. Alexandria, WHO Regional Office for the Eastern Mediterranean (assignment report).

Arfaa F (1988b) *Schistosomiasis control programme in Saudi Arabia*. Alexandria, WHO Regional Office for the Eastern Mediterranean (assignment report, 20 October 1984 to 31 December 1987).

Audibert M (1982) La prévalence de la schistosomiase à *S. haematobium* dans le Mayo Danaï (Nord Cameroun). *Comptes rendus de la 14e Conférence Technique de l'OCEAC*, Yaoundé, pp. 419–429.

Audibert M (1986) Agricultural non-wage production and health status. A case study in a tropical environment. *Journal of development economics*, **24**: 275–291.

Audibert M et al. (1983) Prévalence de la schistosomiase à *Schistosoma haematobium* dans le Mayo Danaï (Nord Cameroun). *Acta tropica*, **40**: 177–186.

Audibert M et al. (1990) Irrigation, schistosomiasis and malaria in the Logone Valley, Cameroon. *American journal of tropical medicine and hygiene*, **42**: 546–549.

Aung Tun Thet (1989) *The Sedawgyi multipurpose dam and irrigation project*. New Delhi, WHO Regional Office for South-East Asia (unpublished document), pp. 122–129.

Awad El Karim MA et al. (1980). Quantitative egg excretion and work capacity in a Gezira population infected with *S. mansoni*. *American journal of tropical medicine and hygiene*, **29**: 54–61.

Bang YH (1988) Vector-borne diseases associated with rice cultivation and their control in South-east Asia. In: *Vector-borne disease control in humans through rice agro-ecosystem management*. Los Baños, Philippines, International Rice Research Institute.

Bang YH, Pant CD (1983) A review on disease vectors breeding in rice fields in tropical Asia and research needs. *Communicable diseases*, **15**: 268–279.

Bani S, Lechuga P, Ridell C (1990) Barrage de retenue d'eau et développement de la schistosomiase. Cas du barrage hydro-électrique de la Kompienga au Burkina Faso. *Actes de la Conférence Internationale OCCGE, Les Schistosomiases*, Niamey, pp. 69–73.

Barbosa LAC (1990) *Availiação da schistossomiase urinaria no canteiro de obras de Capanda*. Terceiro journada de medicina militar, Luanda (unpublished manuscript).

Bassily S et al. (1987) Immunogenicity of hepatitis B vaccine in patients infected with *Schistosoma mansoni*. *American journal of tropical medicine and hygiene*, **36**: 549–553.

Baum WC (1982) *The project cycle*. Washington, DC, World Bank.

Betterton C (1984) Ecological studies on the snail hosts of schistosomiasis in the South Chad Irrigation Project Area, Borno State, northern Nigeria. *Journal of arid environments*, **7**: 43–57.

Betterton C et al. (1988) Schistosomiasis in Kano State, Nigeria. I. Human infection near dam sites and the distribution and habitat preferences of potential snail intermediate hosts. *Annals of tropical medicine and parasitology*, **82**: 561–570.

Birley MH (1989) *Guidelines for forecasting the vector-borne disease implications of water resource development projects*. Geneva, World Health Organization (unpublished document no. VBC/89.6).

Blacklock DB (1924) Report on an investigation into the prevalence and transmission of human schistosomiasis in Sierra Leone. *Annual report of the Medical and Sanitary Department for the year 1923*, Freetown.

Blas B (1976) Agroengineering and sanitation improvement in control of *S. japonica* in the Philippines. In: *Proceedings of the Fourteenth SEAMEO-tropical medicine seminar. Schistosomiasis in South-East Asia and the Far East*, Manila.

Blas B (1989) *The schistosomiasis control programme in the Philippines.* Meeting on the strategy of control of morbidity due to schistosomiasis, Geneva, 10–13 October 1989. Geneva, World Health Organization (unpublished document).

Blue Nile Health Project (1985) A comprehensive approach to the prevention and control of water-associated diseases in irrigated schemes of the Sudan. *Journal of tropical medicine and hygiene*, **88**: 1–182.

Bolton P (1988) *Health issues in irrigation development in Africa: an engineer's perspective.* Wallingford, Hydraulics Research, Overseas Development Unit (unpublished document).

Bradley DJ (1977) The health implications of irrigation schemes and man-made lakes in tropical environments. In: *Water, wastes and health in hot climates*, London, John Wiley & Son, pp. 18–29.

Brasil-Paraguay/Itaipu Binacional (1975) *Hidrelectrica de Itaipu. Plano básico para conservaçao do meio ambiente.* Rio de Janeiro-Assunçao, Itaipu Binacional.

Brasil-Paraguay/Itaipu Binacional (1978) *Estatistica de accidentes* (unpublished document).

Brengues J (1975) *La filariose de Bancroft en Afrique de l'Ouest.* Paris, ORSTOM (Mémoires ORSTOM No. 79).

Breuil J et al. (1983a) Tentatives d'appréciation du retentissement socio-économique des schistosomiases à Madagascar. *Archives de l'Institut Pasteur de Madagascar*, **50**: 97–111.

Breuil J et al. (1983b) Bilan parasitologique d'une population du nord-ouest de Madagascar avant travaux d'aménagement hydraulique pour l'extension d'un complexe sucrier (Ambilobe). *Archives de l'Institut Pasteur de Madagascar*, **50**: 113–119.

Brinkmann UK, Korte R, Schmidt-Ehry B (1988) The distribution and spread of schistosomiasis in relation to water resources development in Mali. *Tropical medicine and parasitology*, **39**: 182–185.

Brinkmann UK et al. (1989) *Schistosomiasis control in Africa: organizational aspects of GTZ-assisted bilateral programmes in Madagascar, Malawi, Mali and the People's Republic of the Congo.* Geneva, World Health Organization (unpublished document no. WHO/SCHISTO/89.100).

Brown DS, Wright CA (1985) Schistosomiasis: bilharzia. In: Grove AT, ed., *The Niger and its neighbours.* Rotterdam, A.A. Balkema, pp. 295–317.

Brown DS et al. (1984) Aquatic snails of the Jonglei region, southern Sudan, and transmission of trematode parasites. *Hydrobiologia*, **110**: 247–271.

Brunet-Jailly J (1982) Riziculture et schistosomiase: une première discussion. *Comptes rendus de la 14e Conférence technique de l'OCEAC*, Yaoundé, pp. 430–436.

Bunnag T, Sornmani S, eds (1989) *The impact of water resources development on the health of the communities and preventive measures for adverse effects. Proceedings of the 13th SEAMEO TROPMED Seminar.* Bangkok, Mahidol University.

Burgis MJ, Morris P (1987) *The natural history of lakes.* Cambridge, Cambridge University Press.

Cairncross S, Feachem RG (1983) *Environmental health engineering in the tropics: an introductory text*. New York, John Wiley & Sons.

Carpenter SR, ed. (1987) *Complex interactions in lake communities*. New York, Springer Verlag.

Centre for Science and Ecology (1982) *India's environment, 1982*. New Delhi.

Centre for Science and Ecology (1985) *India's environment, 1984–1985*. New Delhi.

Chaine JP (1984) *Schistosomiasis prevalence and control in the Kingdom of Swaziland*. Washington, DC, American Public Health Association.

Chandiwana S et al. (1988) Control of schistosomiasis transmission in newly established smallholder irrigation schemes. *Transactions of the Royal Society of Tropical Medicine and Hygiene*, **82**: 874–880.

Chen H-L et al. (1989) [Predictive impact on malaria prevalence of the hydraulic project of Three Gorges of the Yangtze river.] *Chinese journal of parasitology and parasitic diseases*, **7**(3): 177–180 (in Chinese).

Chowdhury AW (1975) Potential effects of irrigation on the spread of bilharziasis in Kenya. *East African medical journal*, **52**: 120–126.

Chowdhury AW (1979) Schistosomiasis control in the Bunyala irrigation scheme—a pilot project in the Yala Swamp of Western Kenya. *East African medical journal*, **56**: 71–75.

Chowdhury AW, Levy BS (1988). *Morbidity estimates of occupational illnesses and injuries in Kenya: human and economic costs*. Unpublished paper presented at the Annual Medical Scientific Conference, Kenya Medical Research Institute—Kenya Tropical Research Institute, Nairobi, 2 February 1988.

Chu KY, Massoud J, Arfaa F (1968) Distribution and ecology of *Bulinus truncatus* in Khuzestan, Iran. *Bulletin of the World Health Organization*, **39**: 607–637.

Chu KY, Klumpp R, Kofi DY (1981) Results of three years of cercarial transmission control in the Volta Lake. *Bulletin of the World Health Organization*, **59**: 549–554.

Clarke JL (1982) *Integrated vector control in the Adana project, Turkey*. Geneva, World Health Organization (unpublished document VBC/ECV/EC/82.11).

Coates D, Redding-Coates TA (1981) Ecological problems associated with irrigation canals in the Sudan with particular reference to the spread of bilharziasis, malaria and aquatic weeds and ameliorative role of fishes. *International journal of environmental studies*, **16** (3/4): 207–212.

CODEVASF (Companhia de Desenvolvimento do Vale do São Francisco) (1989) *Report for 1985–1988*. Brasilia.

Conselho Nacional de Desenvolvimento Cientifico e Technológico (CNPQ) (1979) *Epidemiologia e control de esquistossomose e o nordeste semiárido*. Report of a Working Group, Recife, 24–28 April 1978.

Cooper Weil DE et al. (1990) *The impact of development policies on health. A review of the literature*. Geneva, World Health Organization.

Coosemans M, Barutwanayo M (1989) Malaria control by antivectorial measures in a zone of chloroquine-resistant malaria: a successful programme in a rice-growing area of the Rusizi valley, Burundi. *Transactions of the Royal Society of Tropical Medicine and Hygiene*, **83** (Suppl.): 97–98.

Coosemans M, Mouchet J (1990). Consequences of rural development on vectors and their control. *Annales de la Société belge de Médicine tropicale*, **70**: 5–23.

Coumbaras A, Picot H (1979) *Hydraulic projects and health problems: directives for study, prevention and control*. Geneva, World Health Organization (unpublished document MPD/PDP).

Daffalla AA, Babiker A, El Gaddal AA (1988) *Blue Nile Health Project. Annual report.* Khartoum, Ministry of Health.

Dazo BC, Biles JE (1972) *Schistosomiasis in the Kainji Lake area, Nigeria. Report on a survey made in October–December 1970.* Geneva, World Health Organization (unpublished document WHO/SCHISTO/72.21).

Dazo BC, Biles JE (1973) *Follow-up studies on the epidemiology of schistosomiasis in the Kainji Lake area, Nigeria, November–December 1971.* Geneva, World Health Organization (unpublished document WHO/SCHISTO/73.29).

De Cock K et al. (1982) Esophageal varices in Nairobi, Kenya: a study of 68 cases. *American journal of tropical medicine and hygiene,* **31**: 579–588.

Degremont AA (1973) *Project Mangoky: Lutte contre les schistosomiases dans le Bas-Mangoky (Madagascar).* Basel, Swiss Tropical Institute.

Delbaere M (1989) *A preliminary investigation on schistosomiasis in the northern Ubangi area, Zaire.* Geneva, World Health Organization (unpublished report).

Deschiens R, Cornu M (1976) Commentaires écologiques et épidémiologiques concernant les bilharzioses et le lac de retenue de Kossou (Côte d'Ivoire). *Bulletin de la Société de Pathologie exotique et de ses Filiales (Paris),* **69**: 163–169.

Doumenge JP et al. (1987) *CEGET/WHO atlas of the global distribution of schistosomiasis.* Bordeaux, Presses Universitaires de Bordeaux.

Draper AJ, Bolton P (1986) *Design note for schistosomiasis control: Mushandike Irrigation Scheme, Zimbabwe.* Wallingford, Hydraulics Research, Overseas Development Unit (Hydraulics research report, no. OD/TN 20).

Drijvers CA (1990) The environmental impacts: disaster or development? *The courier,* **124**: 68–69.

Duplantier J et al. (1990) *Rongeurs et dégats des rongeurs.* Dakar, ORSTOM (Programme "Eau, santé et développement", annual report for 1990).

Edungbola LD et al. (1986) The status of human onchocerciasis in the Kainji reservoir basin areas 20 years after the impoundment of the lake. *Tropical and geographical medicine,* **38** (3): 226–232.

Egypt (1987) Report of an independent evaluation mission on the national bilharzia control program in Egypt. *Transactions of the Royal Society of Tropical Medicine and Hygiene,* **81** (Supplement): 1–57.

Eouzan JP (1980) Déplacements de populations et trypanosomiase humaine en Afrique centrale. *Insect science and its application,* **1**: 99–103.

Evans AC (1983) Control of schistosomiasis in large irrigation schemes by use of niclosamide: a ten-year study in Zimbabwe. *American journal of tropical medicine and hygiene,* **32**: 1029–1039.

Fadl OAA (1990) Gezira: the largest irrigation scheme in Africa. *The courier,* **124**, 91–94.

Farid MA (1977) Irrigation and malaria in arid lands. In: Worthington EB, ed. *Arid land irrigation in developing countries. Environmental problems and effects.* Oxford, Pergamon, pp. 413–419.

Fels E, Keller R (1973) World register of man-made lakes. In: Ackermann WC, White GF, Worthington EB, ed. *Man-made lakes: their problems and environmental effects.* Washington, DC, American Geophysical Union, pp. 43–49.

Fenwick A (1989) Irrigation in the Sudan and schistosomiasis. In: Service MW, ed. *Demography and vector-borne diseases,* Boca Raton, FL, CRC Press, pp. 333–351.

Finelle P (1980) Répercussions des programmes d'aménagement hydraulique et rural sur l'épidémiologie et l'épizootologie des trypanosomiases. *Insect science and its application,* **1**: 95–98.

FAO (1987a) *The effects of agricultural development on vector-borne diseases.*

Rome, Food and Agriculture Organization of the United Nations (Joint WHO/FAO/UNEP Panel of Experts on Environmental Management for Vector Control. AGL/MISC/12/87).

FAO (1987b) *Consultation on irrigation in Africa*. Rome, Food and Agriculture Organization of the United Nations (FAO Irrigation and Drainage Paper No. 42).

FAO (1989a) *The state of food and agriculture*. Rome, Food and Agriculture Organization of the United Nations.

FAO (1989b) *Yearbook: production, Volume 43*. Rome, Food and Agriculture Organization of the United Nations.

FAO (1990) Irrigation in Africa: a potential for small units. *The courier*, **124**: 65–67.

FAO/SIDA (Swedish International Development Authority) (1990) *Gender issues in fisheries and aquaculture: including proceedings of the workshop on enhanced women's participation in fisheries development*. Victoria Falls, Zimbabwe, 4-7 December 1990 (document GCP/INT/436/SWE/REP/7).

Fouya AM (1990) Improving small farmer-managed plots. *The courier*, **124**: 76–77.

Futa AB (1983) Water resources development – organisation of a resettlement programme (a case study of the Kpong Resettlement Programme in Ghana). *Water international*, **8** (3): 98–101.

GAMEK (Gabinete de Aproveitamento de Medio Kwanza) (1988) *Natureza e objecto*. Luanda, Angola.

Gani A, Rivany R (1989) Eradication program and related issues of schistosomiasis in Sulewasi, Indonesia. In: *South-East Asia Regional Symposium on the Implication of Public Policy on Health Status and Quality of Life, Bangalore, India, 18–26 October 1989*. New Delhi, WHO Regional Office for South-East Asia (unpublished document).

Ghaffar YA et al. (1990) Hepatitis B vaccination in children infected with *Schistosoma mansoni*: correlation with ultrasound data. *American journal of tropical medicine and hygiene*, **43**: 516–519.

Ghana Health Assessment Project Team (1981) A quantitative method for assessing the health impact of different diseases in less developed countries. *International journal of epidemiology*, **10**: 73–79.

Gigase P, Hanotier J (1982) Bilharziose. In: *Santé et maladies au Rwanda*. Brussels, Administration Générale de la Coopération au Développement.

Giglioli MEC (1979) *Irrigation, anophelism and malaria in Adana, Turkey. An appraisal report on the Seyhan Irrigation Project for the World Bank*. Washington, DC, World Bank (unpublished report).

Gill CA (1930) The relationship of canal irrigation and malaria. *Records of the malaria survey of India*, **1**: 417–421.

Githaiga HK (1983) *Assignment report: schistosomiasis prevention and control in the Sultanate of Oman*. Alexandria, WHO Regional Office for the Eastern Mediterranean (unpublished document no. EM/Schis/85).

Goldsmith E, Hildyard N (1985) *The social and environmental effects of large dams. Vol. 1. Overviews*. Camelford, Cornwall, Wadebridge Ecological Centre.

Goldsmith E, Hildyard N (1986) *The social and environmental effects of large dams. Vol. 2, Case studies*. Camelford, Cornwall, Wadebridge Ecological Centre.

Goodland R (1985) *Environmental aspects of tropical water development projects*. International Seminar on Environmental Impact Assessment of Water Resources projects. University of Roorkee, Uttar Pradesh, India, 12–14 December 1985 (unpublished document).

Goodland R (1989) *The World Bank's new policy on the environmental aspects of dam and reservoir projects.* Washington, DC, World Bank (World Bank Reprint Series, no. 458).

Goodland R et al. (1990) Tropical moist forest management: the urgency of transition to sustainability. *Environmental conservation*, **17**: 303–318.

Graham R (1986) Ghana's Volta Resettlement Scheme. In: Goldsmith E, Hildyard N, eds. *The social and environmental effects of large dams. Vol. 2. Case studies.* Camelford, Cornwall, Wadebridge Ecological Centre, pp. 131–139.

Greer G, Inder Singh K, Lim HK (1980) Discovery of a site of transmission and hosts of a *Schistosoma japonicum*-like schistosome in peninsular Malaysia. *Transactions of the Royal Society of Tropical Medicine and Hygiene*, **74**: 425.

Greer G et al. (1989) Malaysian schistosomiasis: description of a population at risk. *Journal of tropical medicine and hygiene*, **92**: 203–208.

Gryseels B (1990) *The distribution and epidemiology of schistosomiasis in Burundi.* Leiden, University of Leiden (doctoral thesis).

Gu X-G et al. (1988) [*Studies on the impact of the Three Gorges Hydraulic Works of Changjiang (Yangtze River) on the spread of schistosomiasis: a special' report.*] Sichuan, Institute of Parasitic Diseases, Sichuan Provincial Academy of Medical Sciences (in Chinese).

Gunatilleke G, ed. (1985) *Migration of Asian workers to the Arab world.* New York, United Nations University.

Hagi H (1986) *Schistosoma haematobium in Somalia: epidemiological and methodological aspects.* Stockholm, Karolinska Institute (dissertation).

Haight B (1990) Fish from small water bodies. *ALCOM news,* **3**: 9–13.

Haile-Meskal F, Kloos H (1989) Vector-borne disease occurrence and spread as affected by labour migrations to irrigation schemes in Ethiopia. In: Service MW, ed., *Demography and vector-borne diseases.* Boca Raton, FL, CRC Press, pp. 225–236.

Haile-Meskal F et al. (1985) Endemicity of urinary schistosomiasis in Enta-Doyta village, Gewane Flood-Plain, Eastern Ethiopia. *Ethiopian medical journal*, **23**: 107–115.

Hammad A El Bindari, Mulholland CA (1989) *The health status of vulnerable groups: a valuable indicator for national development.* Paper presented at a workshop on Methods of Studying Health Transition Processes, London School of Hygiene and Tropical Medicine, June 1989.

Hazza YA, Arfaa F, Haggar M (1983). Studies on schistosomiasis in Taiz Province, Yemen Arab Republic. *American journal of tropical medicine and hygiene,* **32**: 1023–1028.

Highton RB (1974) Health risks in water conservation schemes. In: Vogel LC, ed. *Health and disease in Kenya.* Nairobi, East African Literature Bureau, pp. 175–178.

Hira PR (1970) Schistosomiasis at Lake Kariba. I. Prevalence and potential intermediate snail hosts at Siavonga. *Tropical and geographical medicine*, **22**: 323–334.

Houston CE (1977). Irrigation development in the world. In: Worthington EB, ed. *Arid land irrigation in developing countries. Environmental problems and effects.* Oxford, Pergamon, pp. 425–432.

Howarth SE et al. (1988) Worms, wells and water in Western Madagascar. *Journal of tropical medicine and hygiene,* **91**: 255–264.

Hubendick B (1958) Factors conditioning the habitat of freshwater snails. *Bulletin of the World Health Organization*, **18**: 1072–1080.

Hughes CC, Hunter JM (1970) Diseases and "development" in Africa. *Social science and medicine*, **3**: 443–493.

Hunter JM (1966) River blindness in Nangodi, northern Ghana: an hypothesis of cyclical advance and retreat. *Geographical review*, **56**: 398–416.

Hunter JM (1967a) Population pressure in a part of the West African savanna: a study of Nangodi, northern Ghana. *Annals of the Association of American Geographers*, **57**: 101–114.

Hunter JM (1967b) Seasonal hunger in a part of the West African savanna: a survey of body weights in Nangodi, north east Ghana. *Transactions, Institute of British Geographers*, **41**: 167–185.

Hunter JM (1981) Past explosion and future threat: exacerbation of red water disease (*Schistosomiasis haematobium*) in the Upper Region of Ghana. *GeoJournal*, **5** (4): 305–313.

Hunter JM (1992) Elephantiasis: a disease of development in northeast Ghana. *Social science and medicine*, **35**: 627–649.

Hunter JM, Rey L, Scott D (1980) *Disease prevention and control in water development schemes.* Geneva, World Health Organization (unpublished document PDP/80.1).

Hunter JM, Rey L, Scott D (1982) Man-made lakes and man-made diseases: towards a policy resolution. *Social science and medicine*, **16**: 1127–1145.

Iarotski LS, Davis A (1981) The schistosomiasis problem in the world: results of a WHO survey. *Bulletin of the World Health Organization*, **59**: 115–127.

Iarotski LS, Pluscheva GL (1989) *Parasitic diseases in water resources development schemes in the USSR.* Moscow, Martsinovsky Institute of Parasitic Diseases (unpublished document).

ICOLD (1973) *World register of dams.* Paris, International Commission on Large Dams.

ICOLD (1974) *World register of dams. First updating.* Paris, International Commission on Large Dams.

ICOLD (1979) *World register of dams. Second updating.* Paris, International Commission on Large Dams.

ICOLD (1985) *World register of dams: full edition 1984.* Paris, International Commission on Large Dams.

ICOLD (1989) *World register of dams: updating 1988.* Paris, International Commission on Large Dams.

Indian Institute of Management (1989) The Narmada Valley Project. In: *South-East Asia Regional Symposium on the Implications of Public Policy on Health Status and Quality of Life, Bangalore, 18–26 October 1989.* New Delhi, WHO Regional Office for South-East Asia (unpublished document).

IRRI (1988) *Vector-borne disease control in humans through rice agroecosystem management.* Manila, International Rice Research Institute.

Isrin I (1989) Schistosomiasis control in Indonesia. In: *WHO meeting on the Strategy of Control of Morbidity due to Schistosomiasis, Geneva, 10–13 October 1989.* Geneva, World Health Organization (unpublished report).

Jannin J et al. (1982) Dépistage de la bilharziose à *S. haematobium* et traitement (Oltipraz) collectif et ambulatoire d'une population de 12000 habitants de la région rizicole de Yagoua (Nord Cameroun). *Comptes rendus de la 14e Conference technique de l'OCEAC*, Yaoundé pp. 461–467.

Jewsbury JM, Imevbore AMA (1988) Small dam health statistics. *Parasitology today*, **4**: 57–58.

Jobin WR (1989) Environmental management measures in water impoundments:

a reservoir study in East Africa (Juba Valley, Somalia). In: *Workshop Proceedings of the WHO Regional Workshop on Environmental Management for Vector Control, Lahore, Pakistan, 7–16 October 1989*, pp. 209–234.

Joubert J et al. (1990) Schistosomiasis of the spinal cord—underdiagnosed in South Africa? *South African medical journal*, **77** (6): 297–299.

Khalil Bey M (1949) The national campaign for the treatment and control of bilharziasis from the scientific and economic aspects. *Journal of the Royal Egyptian Medical Association*, **32**: 820.

Kloos H, Lemma A (1977) Schistosomiasis in irrigation schemes in the Awash Valley. *American journal of tropical medicine and hygiene*, **26**: 899–908.

Klumpp RK, Chu KY (1977) Ecological studies of *Bulinus rohlfsi*, the intermediate host of *Schistosoma haematobium* in the Volta Lake. *Bulletin of the World Health Organization*, **55**: 715–730.

Kuzoe FAS (1973) Entomological aspects of trypanosomiasis at Volta Lake. *Geophysical monograph series*, **17**: 129–131.

Lamothe F et al. (1989) Etude echographique de la morbidité due a la bilhariziose urinaire dans un village hiperendemique nigerien. *Bulletin de la Société de Pathologie exotique et de ses Filiales*, **82**(5): 678–684.

Lanoix JN (1958) Relation between irrigation engineering and bilharziasis. *Bulletin of the World Health Organization*, **18**: 1011–1035.

Latham MC et al. (1990) Metrifonate or praziquantel treatment improves physical fitness and appetite of Kenyan schoolboys with *Schistosoma haematobium* and hookworm infections. *American journal of tropical medicine and hygiene*, **43**: 170–179.

LeBras M et al. (1982) Activités humaines, aménagements hydroagricoles et schistosomiase urinaire. Approche méthodologique et résultats. *Bulletin de la Société de Pathologie exotique*, **75**: 44–54.

LeBerre R (1971) *Le foyer d'onchocercose de Loumana, Cercle de Sindou, Haute Volta.* Bobo-Dioulasso, ORSTOM (unpublished document).

Liese BH, Sachdeva PS, Cochrane DG (1991) *Organizing and managing tropical disease control programs: lessons of success.* Washington, DC, World Bank (Technical Paper No. 154).

Lipton M, de Kadt E (1988) *Agriculture-health linkages.* Geneva, World Health Organization (Offset Publication No. 104).

Lo CT et al. (1989) Schistosomiasis in the Gumara and Ribb Irrigation Project Area, Ethiopia. *Ethiopian medical journal*, **27**: 47–53.

Lockhardt JDF, Highton RB, McMahon JP (1969) Public health problems arising out of man-made fish ponds in the western province of Kenya fish culture. *East African medical journal*, **46**: 471–480.

Logan JWM (1983) Schistosomiasis in Swaziland—a comparative study of three irrigated estates. *Journal of helminthology*, **57**: 247–253.

Lu BL (1984) [*The integrated control of mosquitos.*] Beijing, Scientific Press (in Chinese).

Malek EA (1983) *Impact of fish ponds on public health in Rwanda with special reference to schistosomiasis.* Kigali, USAID (unpublished document).

Malek EA (1985) *Impact of irrigated agriculture on public health in Niger with special reference to schistosomiasis.* Niamey, USAID (unpublished document).

Malek EA, Chaine JP (1989) Effects of the developments in the Senegal River Basin on the prevalence and spread of schistosomiasis. In: Service MW, ed., *Demography and vector-borne diseases.* Boca Raton, FL, CRC Press, pp. 181–192.

Mallett JC, Aboul-Ela IA (1979) A new range of extension of *Biomphalaria alexandrina,* the snail intermediate host of *Schistosoma mansoni* in Egypt. *Malacological reviews,* **12**: 91–92.

Mara D, Cairncross S (1989) *Guidelines for the safe use of wastewater and excreta in agriculture and aquaculture.* Geneva, World Health Organization.

Masaba SC, Ochieng S, Awino MO (1983) Man-made dams acting as sources of bilharziasis in Onganga village, Kanyaluo location, South Nyanza. *East African medical journal,* **60**: 860–862.

Massoud J et al. (1982) Progress in the national schistosomiasis control programme of Iran. *Bulletin of the World Health Organization,* **60**: 577–582.

Mather TH, That TT (1984) *Environmental management for vector control in rice fields.* Rome, Food and Agriculture Organization of the United Nations (Irrigation and Drainage Paper No. 41).

Mather TH, Bos R (1989) *Policies and programs of governments, bilateral and multilateral agencies and development banks for environmental management in the context of natural resources, agriculture and health development.* Geneva, World Health Organization (unpublished document VBC/89.7).

Matovu DB (1978) Prospects of schistosomiasis in the proposed Lake Mtera in Tanzania. *Tropical and geographical medicine,* **30**: 193–197.

Mbulamberi DB (1989) Possible causes leading to an epidemic outbreak of sleeping sickness: facts and hypotheses. *Annales de la Société belge de Médecine tropicale,* **69** (Suppl. 1): 173–179.

McJunkin FE (1975) *Water, engineers, development and disease in the tropics. Schistosomiasis engineering applied to planning, design, construction and operation of irrigation, hydroelectric and other water development schemes.* Washington, DC, United States Agency for International Development.

Meier-Brook C (1974) A snail intermediate host of *Schistosoma mansoni* introduced into Hong Kong. *Bulletin of the World Health Organization,* **51**: 661.

Miller MJ (1981) *Parasites of man and arthropod disease vectors in communities of a water development project on the Senegal River Basin.* Dakar, Senegal (unpublished report to USAID).

Morrow RH (1984) The application of a quantitative approach to the assessment of the relative importance of vector and soil transmitted diseases in Ghana. *Social science and medicine,* **19**: 1039–1049.

Mott KE, Davis A (1986) *Organizational implications of various control programme strategies.* World Bank/WHO/Edna McConnell Clark Foundation Workshop on Organization and Management of Control Programmes for Schistosomiasis and other Endemic Diseases, 9–11 June 1986, Washington, DC.

Mott KE et al. (1986) *A proposed national plan of action for schistosomiasis control in the United Republic of Cameroon.* Geneva, World Health Organization (unpublished document WHO/SCHISTO/86.88).

Mouchet J, Brengues J (1990) Les interfaces agriculture-santé dans les domaines de l'épidémiologie des maladies à vecteurs et de la lutte antivectorielle. *Bulletin de la Société de Pathologie exotique et de ses Filiales,* **83** (3): 376–393.

Muigai RK et al. (1989) Schistosomiasis caused by *Schistosoma mansoni* in Baringo District, Kenya: case report. *East African medical journal,* **66** (10): 700–702.

Mukiama TK, Mwangi RW (1989) Seasonal population changes and malaria transmission potential of *Anopheles pharoensis* and the minor anophelines in Mwea Irrigation Scheme, Kenya. *Acta tropica,* **46**: 181–189.

Mwanza Medical Research Centre (1982) *The prevalence and incidence of schistosomiasis and the projected impact of the development in the lower Rufiji Valley.* Mwanza, National Institute for Medical Research.

Najera JA (1981) Problemas relacionados con modificaciones del medio ambiente y con la ecología humana. In: *Malaria in las Americas*, Washington, DC, Pan American Health Organization (Scientific Publication, No. 405).

Ndamba J (1986) Schistosomiasis: its effects on the physical performance of school-children in Zimbabwe. *Central African journal of medicine*, **32** (12): 289–293.

Ndamba J et al. (1991) Morbidity due to *Schistosoma mansoni* among sugar-cane cutters. *International journal of epidemiology*, **20**: 787–795.

Ngindu AM (1990) Strengthening needs in the planning and management of integrated vector-borne disease control. In: WHO/FAO/UNEP, *Water resources development and vectorborne diseases in Kenya*. Geneva, World Health Organization (unpublished document no. CWS/90.4), pp. 53–56.

N'Goran KE (1987) *Situation épidémiologique des schistsomiases en zone rurale du centre de la Côte d'Ivoire. Influence d'un barrage a vocation agro-pastorale.* National University of Côte d'Ivoire (Thesis No. 109).

Niger (1980) *Marchés tropicaux et méditerranéens*, **35** (1751): 1408.

Noamesi GK, Morcos G (1974) *Health component in South Chad Irrigation Project feasibility study: follow-up studies on schistosomiasis and malaria.* Brazzaville, WHO Regional Office for Africa (unpublished document AFR/SCHIST/30).

Odei MA (1973) Observations on some weeds of malacological importance in the Volta Lake. *Bulletin de l'Institut française d'Afrique noire*, Série A, **35** (1): 57–66.

Odei MA (1977) *Report of the status of the ecology and prevalence of vectors of schistosomiasis and fascioliasis in the area of the second Volta dam at Kpong.* Accra, Institute of Aquatic Biology (IAB) (Technical Report IAB No. 68).

Odei MA (1981) *Survey for the distribution of vector snails and the trematodes of medical and veterinary importance which they transmit in Ghana.* Report to the WHO/UNDP/World Bank Special Programme on Research and Training in Tropical Diseases (SCH) T16/181/B2/20.

Odingo' RS (1965) *Multipurpose river basin development in developing countries. Report of an international workshop.* Nairobi, Department of Geography, University of Nairobi.

Ohse T (1980) *Rapport de mission pour l'aménagement et le développement du bassin de la rivière Kagera.* Kigali, World Health Organization (unpublished document).

Omer AHS (1978). Schistosomiasis in the Sudan: historical background and the present magnitude of the problem. In: *Proceedings of the International Conference on Schistosomiasis, Cairo, 1975*, Cairo, Ministry of Health, Vol. 1, pp. 121–132.

OMVS (1992) (Organization pour la Mise en Valeur de la Vallée du Fleuve Sénégal) *Evaluation des effets sur l'environnement d'aménagements prévus dans le bassin du fleuve Sénégal. Rapport spécial Bilharziose.* Narrisburg, Pennsylvania, Garnett Fleming Corddry and Carpenter Inc.

Onori E et al. (1963) Schistosomiasis in the Volta region of Ghana. *Annals of tropical medicine and parasitology*, **57**: 59–67.

Oomen JMV (1981) *Monitoring health in African dams: the Kamburu Dam (Kenya) as a test case.* University of Rotterdam (thesis).

Oomen JMV, de Wolf J, Jobin W (1988) *Health and irrigation.* Wageningen, Netherlands, International Land Reclamation Institute (publication 45, volume 2).

Oomen JMV, de Wolf J, Jobin W (1990) *Health and irrigation.* Wageningen, Netherlands, International Land Reclamation Institute (publication 45, volume 1).

Oostberg BFJ (1977) *Brokopondo, Kabalebo and health care.* In: Panday RS, ed.,

Man-made lakes and human health. Proceedings of a symposium, Paramaribo 23–25 October 1977. Paramaribo, University of Suriname and Alcoa Foundation. pp. 47–51.

PAHO (1977) *Impactos de la construcción de la presa de Itaipu sobre la salud pública en Paraguay.* Washington, DC, Pan American Health Organization (Report of a Study Group).

PAHO (1990a) *Status of malaria programs in the Americas: XXXVIII report.* Washington, DC, Pan American Health Organization (XXIII Pan American Sanitary Conference: unpublished document no. CSP23/INF/2).

PAHO (1990b) *Health conditions in the Americas. Vol. 1.* Washington, DC, Pan American Health Organization (Scientific Publication No. 524).

Paperna I (1969) Aquatic weeds, snails and transmission of bilharzia in the new man-made Volta Lake in Ghana. *Bulletin de l'Institut français d'Afrique noire,* **31**, Série A (2): 487–499.

Paperna I (1970) Study of an outbreak of schistosomiasis in the newly formed Volta Lake in Ghana. *Zeitschrift für Tropenmedizinische und Parasitologie,* **21**: 411–425.

Pawlowski ZS, Schad GA, Stott GS (1991) *Hookworm infection and anaemia. Approaches to prevention and control.* Geneva, World Health Organization.

Payne AI (1986) *The ecology of tropical lakes and rivers.* Chichester, John Wiley & Sons.

Pereira da Costa DP, Barbosa FS (1985) A esquistossomose e o Nordeste semi-arido. I. O estudo preliminar. *Cadernos de saúde pública, Rio de Janeiro,* **1** (2): 153–159.

Pickford J (1989) *Developing world water.* Hong Kong, Grosvenor Press International.

Pike EG (1987) *Engineering against schistosomiasis/bilharzia. Guidelines towards control of the disease.* London and Basingstoke, Macmillan.

Polderman AM (1984). Cost-effectiveness of different ways of controlling intestinal schistosomiasis: a case study. *Social science and medicine,* **19** (10): 1073–1080.

Pretorius SJ, Joubert PH, de Kock KN (1989). A review of the schistosomiasis risk in South African dams. *Water SA,* **15** (2): 133–136.

Pugh RNH, Gilles HM (1978). Malumfashi Endemic Diseases Research Project, III: Urinary schistosomiasis—a longitudinal study. *Annals of tropical medicine and parasitology,* **72**: 471–482.

Quélennec G, Simonkovitch E, Ovazza M (1968). Recherche d'un type de deversoir de barrage défavorable a l'implantation de *Simulium damnosum* (Diptera, Simuliidae). *Bulletin of the World Health Organization,* **38**: 943–956.

Rajagopalan PK et al. (1990) Parasitological aspects of malaria persistence in Koraput district, Orissa, India. *Indian journal of medical research,* **91**: 44–51.

Rao BA (1945) Malaria in the Irwin Canal area in Mysore Estate. Part I. *Journal of the Malariology Institute of India,* **6**: 101–108.

Rey L (1978) *Report on a travel to South America to visit man-made lakes in Brazil, and to establish preliminary contacts to prepare a seminar on health environment and development in projects for water resources utilization to be held in Argentina or Uruguay.* Geneva, World Health Organization (unpublished document).

Rey L (1979) *Second visit to Jordan to assist national authorities in the prevention of schistosomiasis (mollusc control).* Geneva, World Health Organization (unpublished document EM/SCHIS/75).

Ripert C (1984) Zur Epidemiologie der Darm und Harnwegsbilharziose in den Mandara-Bergen von Nordkamerun. *Medizin in den Entwicklungsländern,* **16**: 169–173.

Ripert C, Raccurt CP (1987). The impact of small dams on parasitic diseases in Cameroon. *Parasitology today*, **3** (9): 287–289.

Ripert C et al. (1979) Évaluation des répercussions sur les endémies parasitaires (malaria, bilharziose, onchocercose, dracunculose) de la construction de 57 barrages dans les Monts Mandara (Nord-Cameroun). *Bulletin de la Société de Pathologie exotique*, **72**: 324–339.

Robert CF et al. (1989) Epidemiology of schistosomiasis in the riverine population of Lagdo Lake, Northern Cameroon: mixed infections. *Tropical medicine and parasitology*, **40**: 153–158.

Robert V et al. (1985) La transmission du paludisme en zone de savane arborée et en zone rizicole des environs de Bobo Dioulasso (Burkina Faso). *Annales de la Société belge de Médecine tropicale*, **65** (Suppl. 2): 201–214.

Roche B et al. (1987) Bilan de cinq années de prospections sur les principales affections parasitaires des Monts Mandara (Nord Cameroun) en rapport avec la construction de barrages et l'aménagement de puits. *Annales universitaires des sciences de la santé (Yaoundé)*, **4** (2): 424–433.

Rollinson D, Simpson AJG, ed. (1987) *The biology of schistosomes. From genes to latrines*. London, Academic Press.

Roundy RW (1989) Problems of resettlement and vector-borne diseases associated with dams and other development schemes. In: Service MW, ed., *Demography and vector-borne diseases*. Boca Raton, FL, CRC Press, pp. 193–205.

Rubin N, Warren WM, ed. (1968) *Dams in Africa. An interdisciplinary study of man-made lakes in Africa*. London, F. Cass & Co.

Russell PF et al. (1940) On the intermittent irrigation of rice fields to control malaria in South India. *Journal of the Malaria Institute of India*, **4**: 321–340.

Saliba EK, Abdel Hafez SK, Tawfiq MR (1986). Schistosomiasis in Jordan: an unwelcome guest. *Parasitology today*, **2**: 91–93.

Samarasinghe MULP (1986) The present malaria situation in Sri Lanka with particular reference to areas where irrigation has recently been introduced. In: *Proceedings of the Workshop on Irrigation and Vector-Borne Disease Transmission*. Sri Lanka, WHO/FAO/UNEP Panel of Experts on Environmental Management for Vector Control, International Irrigation Management Institute.

Sanecki MJ, Diamant BZ (1967) *Health aspects of reclamation of the Yala swamp*. Brazzaville, WHO Regional Office for Africa (unpublished document AFR/CD/14, AFR/FM/69).

Schistosomiasis Symposium (1979) *Schistosomiasis in Egypt. Changing epidemiologic patterns and their implications for control and containment*. Cairo, Ministry of Health.

Schorr TS (1984) *Las represas y sus efectos sobre la salud*. Mexico, Centro Panamericano de Ecología Humana y Salud, Pan American Health Organization (ECO Guía 1).

Schramm G, Warford JJ (1989) *Environmental management and economic development*. Baltimore, Johns Hopkins University Press.

Scott D, Chu KY (1977) *Schistosomiasis research project on man-made lakes. Visit from the project to Mali, 16–29 September 1977*. Geneva, World Health Organization (unpublished document IR/MPD/028).

Sellin B et al. (1983a) Aménagements hydroagricoles et schistosomiase au Niger: recherche d'une méthode de lutte. In: *L'épidémiologie à la géographie humaine*. Bordeaux, Centre d'Etudes de Géographie Tropicale (Travaux et Documents de Géographie Tropicale No. 48), pp. 215–271.

Sellin B et al. (1983b) *Situation épidémiologique de la schistosomiase à Schistosoma haematobium dans la zone du périmètre irrigué rizicole de Liboré, Niger. Pré-*

sentation de la zone et résultats des enquêtes parasitologiques chez l'homme. Niamey, OCCGE, CERMES (report no. I/83).

Sellin B, Simonkovich E (1983) Schistosomiases et barrages en Côte d'Ivoire. In: *L'épidémiologie à la géographie humaine.* Bordeaux, Centre d'Etudes de Géographie Tropicale (Travaux et Documents de Géographie Tropicale No. 48), pp. 209–211.

Service MW, ed (1989a) *Demography and vector-borne diseases.* Boca Raton, FL, CRC Press.

Service MW (1989b) Irrigation: boon or bane? In: Service MW, ed., *Demography and vector-borne diseases.* Boca Raton, FL, CRC Press, pp. 237–254.

Singh N, Singh OP, Soan V (1989) Mosquito breeding in rice fields and its role in malaria transmission in Mandela district, Madhya Pradesh. *Indian journal of malariology,* **26** (4): 191–198.

Sornmani S, Harinasuta C (1988). *Water resources development and its impact on socioeconomics and health with reference to Thailand.* Bangkok, Faculty of Tropical Medicine, Mahidol University.

Southgate VR (1984) The Jonglei canal, Sudan and schistosomiasis. *Biannual report of the British Museum, 1981–1983.* London, British Museum, pp. 68–72.

Southgate VR, Agrawal MC (1990) Human schistosomiasis in India. *Parasitology today,* **6**: 166–168.

Stanley NF, Alpers MP, ed. (1975) *Man-made lakes and human health.* London and New York, Academic Press.

Strickland GT (1982) Providing health services on the Aswan High Dam. *World health forum,* **3**: 297–300.

SUCAM (1976) *Situação de saude na area de influencia da hidrelectrica de Itaipu.* Brazil, Ministry of Health (unpublished document).

Surtees G (1970) Large-scale irrigation and arbovirus epidemiology, Kano Plain, Kenya. Description of the area and preliminary studies on the mosquitoes. *Journal of medical entomology,* **7**: 509–517.

Surtees G (1975) Mosquitoes, arboviruses and vertebrates. In: Stanley NF, Alpers MP, ed. *Man-made lakes and human health.* London and New York, Academic Press, pp. 21–23.

Taha AZ, Merghani OA (1990) Community health in a rural area of Sudan. *Journal of community health,* **15** (4): 267–274.

Taib A (1989) Socioeconomic implication of water resource development projects and their impact on human health with particular reference to the proposed Nenggiri Dam. In: Bunnag T, Sornmani S, *The impact of water resources development on the health of the communities and preventive measures for adverse effects. Proceedings of the 13th SEAMEO TROPMED Seminar.* Bangkok, Mahidol University, pp. 299–311.

Talla I et al. (1990) Outbreak of intestinal schistosomiasis in the Senegal River Basin. *Annales de la Société belge de la Médicine tropicale,* **70**: 173–180.

Taylor P, Makura O (1985) Prevalence and distribution of schistosomiasis in Zimbabwe. *Annals of tropical medicine and parasitology,* **79** (2): 287–299.

Tayo MA, Jewsbury J (1978) Malumfashi Endemic Diseases Research Project, IV. Changes in snail population following the construction of a small dam. *Annals of tropical medicine and parasitology,* **72**: 483–487.

Tech CL (1984) Institutional arrangements of implementation in water resources development project in the Philippines. *Joint WHO/FAO/UNEP Panel of Experts on Environmental Management for Vector Control. Fourth Annual Meeting, Geneva, 1–5 October 1984.* Geneva, World Health Organization (unpublished document no. EPO/PE/WP/84.3).

Tedla S, Kloos H, Tialhun G (1989) *Schistosomiasis in Ethiopia*. Addis Ababa, Addis Ababa University Press.

Teklehaimanot A, Fletcher M (1990) A parasitological and malacological survey of schistosomiasis mansoni in the Beles Valley, northwestern Ethiopia. *Journal of tropical medicine and hygiene*, **93** (1): 12–21.

Tiffen M (1989) *Guidelines for the incorporation of health safeguards into irrigation projects through intersectoral cooperation with special reference to vector-borne diseases*. Geneva, World Health Organization (unpublished document VBC/89.5).

Traore M (1989) Schistosomiasis in the Selingué dam area: the integrated approach. *Tropical medicine and parasitology*, **40**: 228–231.

Trape B et al. (1991) Tick-borne borrelosis in west Africa. *Lancet*, **337**: 473–475.

Umenai T et al. (1985) Japanese encephalitis: current world-wide status. *Bulletin of the World Health Organization*, **63** (4): 625–631.

UNDP/WHO (1979) *Research on the epidemiology and methodology of schistosomiasis control in man-made lakes (RAF/71/217)—Ghana and Egypt. Project findings and recommendations*. Geneva, World Health Organization (unpublished document PDP/79.2).

UNEP (1982) *The state of the environment 1972–1982*. Nairobi, United Nations Environment Programme.

UNEP (1986) *The state of the environment 1986—Environment and health*. Nairobi, United Nations Environment Programme.

UNEP (1987a) *The state of the environment 1987—The state of the world environment*. Nairobi, United Nations Environment Programme.

UNEP (1987b) *Environmental data report*. Oxford, Basil Blackwell.

UNEP (1988) *The state of the environment 1988—the public and environment*. Nairobi, United Nations Environment Programme.

UNEP (1989) *The state of the environment 1989—The state of the world environment*. Nairobi, United Nations Environment Programme.

UNEP (1990) *The state of the environment 1990—children and the environment*. Nairobi, United Nations Environment Programme.

Van Der Lingen MI (1973) Lake Kariba: early history and South Shore. In: Ackermann WC, White GF, Worthington EB, *Man-made lakes: their problems and environmental effects*. Washington, DC, American Geophysical Union (Geophysical Monograph Series, No. 17), pp. 132–169.

Van Ee JH, Polderman AM (1984) Physiological performance and work capacity of tin mine labourers infested with schistosomiasis in Zaire. *Tropical and geographical medicine*, **36**: 259–266.

Vercruysse J, Southgate VR, Rollinson D (1985) The epidemiology of human and animal schistosomiasis in the Senegal River Basin. *Acta tropica*, **42** (3): 249–259.

Vogel LC et al. (1974) *Health and disease in Kenya*. Nairobi, East African Literature Bureau.

Volta River Authority (1977) *The Kpong hydro-power dam*. Unpublished document.

Waddy BB (1972) *Health component in the Kainji Lake Research Project*. Geneva, World Health Organization (unpublished document WHO/AJR/PHA/102).

Waiyaki P (1987) *The history of irrigation development in Kenya and the associated spread of schistosomiasis*. (WHO/FAO/UNEP unpublished document, PEEM/7/WP/87.6a).

Walker J (1978) The finding of *Biomphalaria straminea* amongst fish imported into

Australia. Geneva, World Health Organization (unpublished document WHO/SCHISTO/78.46).

Watson JM (1958) Ecology and distribution of *Bulinus truncatus* in the Middle East. *Bulletin of the World Health Organization*, **18**: 833–894.

Webbe G, El-Hak S (1990) Progress in the control of schistosomiasis in Egypt 1985–1988. *Transactions of the Royal Society of Tropical Medicine and Hygiene*, **84**: 394–400.

Wen ST, Chu KY (1984) Preliminary schistosomiasis survey in the lower Volta River below Akosombo Dam, Ghana. *Annals of tropical medicine and parasitology*, **78**: 129–133.

White GF, ed. (1978) *Environmental effects of arid land irrigation in developing countries*. Paris, United Nations Educational, Scientific and Cultural Organization (Man and the biosphere, Technical Notes 8).

White PT, Coleman M, Jupp BP (1982) Swamp rice development, schistosomiasis and onchocerciasis in southeast Sierra Leone. *American journal of tropical medicine and hygiene*, **31**: 490–498.

White PT, Gbakima AA, Amara SV (1989) *Schistosoma mansoni* in Sierra Leone: an invader extending its range? *Annals of tropical medicine and parasitology*, **83**: 191–193.

WHO (1984) *Lymphatic filariasis*: fourth report of the WHO Expert Committee on Filariasis. Geneva, World Health Organization (WHO Technical Report Series No. 702).

WHO (1985) *The control of schistosomiasis:* report of a WHO Expert Committee. Geneva, World Health Organization (WHO Technical Report Series No. 728).

WHO (1986a) *Intersectoral action for health. The role of intersectoral cooperation in national strategies for health for all*. Geneva, World Health Organization.

WHO (1986b) *Epidemiology and control of African trypanosomiasis*. Geneva, World Health Organization (WHO Technical Report Series No. 739).

WHO (1986c) *WHO Expert Committee on Malaria:* eighteenth report. Geneva, World Health Organization (WHO Technical Report Series No. 735).

WHO (1987a) *WHO Expert Committee on Onchocerciasis*. Geneva, World Health Organization (WHO Technical Report Series No. 752).

WHO (1987b) Schistosomiasis—an unwelcome guest. *Weekly epidemiological record*, **62**: 122–123.

WHO (1987c) *Prevention and control of intestinal parasitic infections*. Geneva, World Health Organization (WHO Technical Report Series No. 749).

WHO (1987d) *Control of lymphatic filariasis. A manual for health personnel*. Geneva, World Health Organization.

WHO (1988) Schistosomiasis control [China]. *Weekly epidemiological record*, **63**: 42–44.

WHO (1989a) *Informal meeting on the global strategy for control of morbidity due to schistosomiasis, Geneva, 10–13 October 1989*. Geneva, World Health Organization (unpublished report no. PDP/SCH).

WHO (1989b) *Progress in assessment of morbidity due to schistosomiasis: reviews of recent literature. Schistosoma haematobium, Schistosoma intercalatum, Schistosoma japonicum, Schistosoma mansoni*. Geneva, World Health Organization (unpublished document).

WHO (1990) *Control of the leishmaniases: report of a WHO Expert Committee*. Geneva, World Health Organization (WHO Technical Report Series No. 793).

WHO (1991) *An overview of the Onchocerciasis Control Programme in West Africa (OCP), 1990.* Geneva, World Health Organization (unpublished document).

WHO (1992a) *Our planet, our health. Report of the WHO Commission on Health and Environment.* Geneva, World Health Organization.

WHO (1992b) *Lymphatic filariasis: the disease and its control: fifth report of the WHO Expert Committee on Filariasis.* Geneva, World Health Organization (WHO Technical Report Series No. 821).

WHO (1993) *The control of schistosomiasis: second report of the WHO Expert Committee.* Geneva, World Health Organization (WHO Technical Report Series No. 830).

WHO Regional Office for Europe (1983) *Environmental health impact assessment of irrigated agricultural development projects: guidelines and recommendations: final report.* London, Environmental Resources Limited.

WHO Regional Office for South-East Asia (1989) *Implications of public policy on health status and quality of life.* New Delhi.

WHO/FAO/UNEP (1986) *Panel of Experts on Environmental Management for Vector Control (PEEM). Report of Sixth Meeting.* Geneva, World Health Organization (unpublished document).

WHO/FAO/UNEP (1987a) PEEM. *Effects of agricultural development on vector-borne diseases.* Rome, Food and Agriculture Organization of the United Nations (unpublished document no. AGL/MISC/12/87).

WHO/FAO/UNEP (1987b) *Selected working papers prepared for the 3rd, 4th, 5th, and 6th meeting of the WHO/FAO/UNEP Panel of Experts on Environmental Management for Vector Control.* Geneva, World Health Organization (unpublished document no. VBC/87.3).

WHO/FAO/UNEP (1990) *Water resources development and vector-borne diseases in Kenya.* Geneva, World Health Organization (unpublished document no. CWS/90.4).

WHO/UNEP (1990) *Public health impact of pesticides used in agriculture.* Geneva, World Health Organization.

Wijesundera M de S (1988) Malaria outbreaks in new foci in Sri Lanka. *Parasitology today,* **4**: 147–150.

World Bank (1987) *Workshop on assessment of human health risks in irrigation and water resource development projects, Paris, 27–28 July 1987.* Washington, DC, World Bank.

World Bank (1989) *World Bank operational manual.* (Operational Directive 4.00, Annex A: Environmental Assessment.) Washington, DC, World Bank).

World Bank/International Monetary Fund (1987) *Environment, growth and development.* Washington, DC, World Bank (Development Committee Publication No. 14).

World Bank/International Monetary Fund (1988) *Environment and development: implementing the World Bank's new policies.* Washington, DC, World Bank (Development Committee Publication No. 17).

World Bank/International Monetary Fund (1989) *World Bank support for the environment: a progress report.* Washington, DC, World Bank (Development Committee Publication No. 22).

World Bank Joint Mission (1985) *Assessment of the risk of introduction of schistosomiasis in water resources development projects and a survey of schistosomiasis in Gimvi, Rathnagiri District, Maharashtra State, India, 13–22 November 1985.* Geneva, World Health Organization (unpublished document).

World Commission on Environment and Development (1987) *Our common future.* Oxford, Oxford University Press.

World Resources Institute (1987) *World resources 1987.* New York, Basic Books.

Worthington EB, ed. (1977) *Arid land irrigation in developing countries. Environmental problems and effects.* Oxford, Pergamon.

Zijlmans CWR et al. (1989) Blaasschistosomiasis bij schoolkinderen; keuzeonderzoek in het Ketudistrict, Ghana. *Nederlands tijdschrift geneeskunde,* **133**: 2552–2556.

Zumstein A (1983) A study of some of the factors influencing the epidemiology of urinary schistosomiasis at Ifakara (Kilombero District, Morogoro Region, Tanzania). *Acta tropica,* **40**: 187–204.

Note: An extensive bibliography on water resources development and health up to 1982 is available from the Documentation and Information Unit of the Division of Control of Tropical Diseases, World Health Organization, 1211 Geneva 27, Switzerland (unpublished document PDP 82.2).

Annex

Suggested technical components of the project health plan and its implementation

Survey and analysis

1. Review of existing health care infrastructure, staff, resources and adaptability in the light of proposed project needs.
2. Survey methodology for endemic human diseases in the area to be affected.
3. Survey methodology for intermediate snail hosts and arthropod vectors and their levels of infectivity in the area to be affected.
4. Methodology to assess the development and anticipated increase or decrease of identified health risks.

Intervention strategy

5. Identification of priority features of the health plan. The strategy may range from no action to be taken, through minimal increased support for existing health care facilities, to varied, targeted or other special chemotherapy programmes and, if required, to a major, coordinated, integrated containment plan. Either vertical or horizontal planning components, involving the local primary health care system, may be required.

Treatment of patients

6. Procurement, distribution and maintenance of essential drugs with appropriate supplementation for schistosomiasis and other water-related diseases (e.g., filariasis, malaria).
7. Training of all health staff to use WHO-recommended treatment schedules for waterborne parasitic diseases.
8. Availability of trained health staff and adequate laboratory facilities for the examination of stool, urine and blood samples with simplified technology for the diagnosis of parasitic diseases.

Recruitment and training of health personnel

9. Identification and training of project supervisors.
10. Recruitment and training of additional nurses and nurse-assistants.
11. Recruitment and training of lay health workers, village programme assistants, paraprofessional/technical labourers (e.g., snail collectors); community mobilization.

Vector control

12. Molluscicidal treatments: different levels, applications and strategies; focal and general; coordinated with treatment of patients. Provision of chemical and other supplies. Pesticide supplies; application regimens.
13. Physical design, engineering, water discipline, channel cleaning and other snail-reducing practices.

Long-term monitoring

14. To avoid the resurgence of disease in communities, or other un-welcome (e.g., vector-related) destabilizations, regular monitoring systems, integrated into the general health care system, should be established. The simplest and most cost-effective approach is to monitor data from peripheral health units. These provide early indications of changes needed for good programme management. An integrated system of appropriate low-cost technology can be established, e.g., involving the use of bicycle couriers. Such a system is more service-able and institutionally long-lasting if established as an incorporated, mainstream activity of the health project structure rather than as a separate institutional appendage.
15. Identification of simple, low-cost technology using:
    — sentinel snails;
    — sentinel mice;
    — chemical reagent strips;
    — indicator houses in villages;
    — indicator work-risk individuals;
    — a flag-alert reporting system in patients' records at clinics.

Improvements in water supply and sanitation

16. Introduction of partially or fully protected water supplies, such as wells, boreholes, pipes, pumps, siphons and adapted natural sites.
17. Introduction of latrines of varied designs, both household and collective; project- and village-sited latrines; distribution of concrete slabs.

Public education, teacher training and continuing education

18. Modification of curricula to promote healthy behaviour and personal hygiene particularly in village primary schools; in-service teacher-training courses and provision of curricular materials on disease prevention and risk avoidance; intersectoral cooperation with ministries of education.

19. Adult education, non-formal village education programmes on disease treatment and prevention; intersectoral cooperation between government agencies; preparation of educational materials, training of instructors (social innovators, change-agents).

Mobilization of village and family support for health

20. Suggestions on utilization of village-level political groups to support health protection. In certain countries, local party cells can serve this purpose.

21. Provision of information and solicitation of support for public health from wider community, district and regional political organizations; lobbying associated with the supplying of information.

22. Suggestions on the marshalling of support for health protection at executive and ministerial levels; understanding, cooperation, and cost- and benefit-sharing in an institutional milieu of intersectoralism.

Index